Praise

Finally, an extremely useful resource for patients that addresses both the physical and emotional health of couples trying to get pregnant! Readers will walk away from each short chapter with action steps they can start today to help support their dream to conceive. I can't wait to recommend this to my patients!

Dr. Joanna Thiessen ND

After trying to conceive for 3 years I read Preconceived and was able to work with my Naturopathic doctor to correct some deficiencies and imbalances. Three months later I finally conceived my son who is now 6 months old and thriving. I would highly recommend this resource to anyone thinking about having a family.

Sarah S. Oakville

A must read, step-by-step guide for anyone on the journey to creating a family. This powerful tool will give you some control and hope during a time many couples and individuals can be fraught with pressure and uncertainty. Preconceived, clearly outlines, what you can do on a daily basis to optimize your health and turn your fertility dreams into reality.

Dr. Olivia Rose ND

PRECONCEIVED

A STEP-BY-STEP GUIDE TO ENHANCING YOUR FERTILITY AND PREPARING YOUR BODY FOR A HEALTHY BABY.

DR. JODIE PEACOCK ND

Copyright © 2020 Jodie Peacock
All rights reserved.

Printed in the United States of America

Published by Author Academy Elite
P.O. Box 43, Powell, OH 43035
www.AuthorAcademyElite.com

All rights reserved. No part of this publication may be reproduced, stored in a retrieval system, or transmitted in any form or by any means—for example, electronic, photocopy, recording—without the prior written permission of the publisher. The only exception is brief quotations in printed reviews.

Paperback ISBN-13: 978-1-64085-513-7
Hardcover ISBN-13: 978-1-64085-514-4

Library of Congress Control Number: 2018967038

Dedicated to my amazing family Chris, Maddox, Cooper and Carter thanks for all your love and support.

TABLE OF CONTENTS

Chapter 1	Introduction	1
Chapter 2	Hormonal Health	4
Chapter 3	Basics of Supplementation	12
Chapter 4	Screening Labs	22
Chapter 5	The Impact of Stress and the Importance of Exercise	32
Chapter 6	The Importance of Sleep	39
Chapter 7	Are eating Organic and Non-GMO Foods important?	45
Chapter 8	The Importance of Fats	54
Chapter 9	Carbohydrates Are Not the Enemy	60
Chapter 10	The Importance of Protein	68

Chapter 11   The Benefits of Smoothies............72

Chapter 12   How to Improve Egg/Oocyte Quality....77

Chapter 13   Optimizing Sperm Health.............86

Chapter 14   The Power of Positive Thought
             and Visualization 97

Chapter 15   Staying Connected and Overcoming
             Strain on Relationships..............105

Chapter 16   The Role of Hormone-Disrupting
             Toxins in Fertility.................110

Chapter 17   Genes and Fertility 117

Final Thoughts 125

Endnotes 127

About the Author 133

ACKNOWLEDGMENTS

Huge thanks to my editorial team Susan, AJ, Joanna and Dave for their editorial excellence

Thanks to Jo, Olivia, Joanne, Lana and the naturopathic community of doctors for the kindness and support.

Shout out to team Paradise, Meredith and Josh for assistance with cover design selection

Thanks to my Mom, Rich, Dave and Keri for your support in all my endeavours.

Thank you to Kary Oberbruner and the team at Author Academy Elite for all your guidance which helped make this book possible.

Thank you always to my husband and boys for allowing me the time to write this book.

CHAPTER 1
INTRODUCTION

I WOULD LIKE to start by congratulating you for wanting to take charge of your health and fertility. This is the first and most important step to improving your health and the health of your soon-to-be-conceived baby.

Today's generation of children is the first in human history that cannot expect to have a longer total life expectancy than their parents. Our world has become more toxic and our food less nutritious, and our bodies aren't evolving quickly enough to keep up with these environmental changes. As a potential mother or father what can you do to reverse this trend? In this book, you will learn the optimal diet, as well as other important lifestyle changes that you can make to optimize your health, enhance your detoxification pathways, and boost your immune system before you conceive. This will go a long way toward improving the health of your eggs or sperm and, therefore, the health of your children. The health-improving process described in this book should ideally start at least three months before you conceive in order to achieve maximum benefit for your baby's health.

I have been a practicing naturopathic doctor in Canada since 2006. My approach to fertility incorporates research-based natural approaches to treating the whole person, rather than just the person's symptoms. In my clinical practice, I work with men, women and couples on their journey to becoming parents. Drawing on my passion for fertility and hormone health, I stress to my patients that preconception is the most crucial time for ensuring the health of their future children.

I have found that there is a vast amount of inaccurate and misleading information about fertility on the Internet. Therefore, I strive to educate couples with research-based natural techniques that will improve both their chance of conception and their overall health. Whether you are just beginning to think about starting a family or have been trying to do so for years, my goal is for you to obtain valuable, scientifically accurate information that can be incorporated into your daily life. Everything in this book can help improve your body's health and prepare you for a healthy conception and pregnancy. The steps I describe can work well on their own or alongside the protocols presented at fertility clinics.

My passion for hormonal health stems from my own personal experience. I was diagnosed with polycystic ovarian syndrome (PCOS) in my early 20s, while I was at school studying to become a naturopathic doctor. I was advised at that time to not wait long to start a family, because most women with PCOS struggle with fertility. However, as I was still in naturopathic medical school, I wasn't quite ready to start a family. I decided instead to dedicate myself to learning everything I could about how to manage hormonal health and optimize fertility naturally—by improving my dietary and lifestyle choices. By following these dietary and lifestyle changes—reflected in the recommendations in this book—I

INTRODUCTION

am proud to say that I was able to conceive my first son and then my twin boys naturally.

After reading *Preconceived*, you will gain knowledge of the following:

- A clear action plan of optimal foods in your diet
- The nutrients/vitamins that are essential for optimizing your health during preconception
- Minimizing exposure to common toxins that can impact conception and health
- Hormonal regulation and the role that stress can play in conception
- Preparing your body for assisted reproductive technologies, such as in vitro fertilization (IVF), to improve the chances of pregnancy
- Appropriate laboratory work that should be performed before you become pregnant, with optimal ranges for healthy conception

This book will empower you to:

- Take control of your health and fertility
- Understand that your diet and lifestyle choices have significant impacts on your baby's health
- Explain that research-based natural treatment has been shown to improve conception and health outcomes
- Implement the take-home information at the end of each chapter

CHAPTER 2
HORMONAL HEALTH

PATIENTS WITH WHOM I have worked over the years have come to me at various points during their fertility journeys. Some are merely considering what they should do to prepare for pregnancy, while others have been trying for many years to conceive. This chapter lays the foundation for a solid understanding of the hormones that are involved in monthly menstrual cycles. This information will reveal how your hormones work to control egg development, ovulation, and uterine lining growth. The association of these processes with overall health will be made clear.

It is important to understand the role that each hormone plays in your body to know when you need to seek the advice of a medical professional. Once you start paying attention to the hormonal signs that your body is giving you, you will be better able to understand what optimal health looks and feels like, and your chances at achieving pregnancy will be enhanced.

At the end of this chapter, you will be able to:

- Name the hormones involved in female reproduction
- Understand how to monitor your menstrual cycle
- Time intercourse based on your cycle monitoring
- Understand how to identify potential problems with your menstrual cycle

Follicle-Stimulating Hormone (FSH)

FOLLICLE-STIMULATING HORMONE (FSH) is released from the pituitary gland in the brain. It stimulates the maturity of the ovarian follicles, which are fluid-filled sacs in the ovary that each contain an immature ovum (egg cell). As the ovarian follicle matures, so does the egg. FSH levels become extremely high when a woman reaches menopause, but levels of this hormone can also fluctuate in younger women. If you have had blood work showing a single high FSH reading, you do not need to panic. Try measuring it again in a subsequent cycle. If the FSH level is consistently elevated, this can be an indicator that your egg reserve is low or that the eggs are not of good quality.

Luteinizing Hormone (LH)

Luteinizing hormone (LH) is released from the pituitary gland at ovulation. It causes the rupture of the mature ovarian follicle, releasing the mature egg.

Estrogen

Estrogen is one of the female sex hormones. It is often referred to as the "growing hormone" because of its role in body development during female puberty. Estrogen is partly responsible for the development of the uterine lining in preparation for implantation of the early embryo. If implantation does not occur, this lining is shed during menstruation. Estrogen also plays a role in maturity of the egg prior to ovulation. Estrogen is produced mostly by the ovaries, but it is also produced in smaller amounts by the adrenal glands and in adipose (fat) tissue. It is the predominant hormone during the first half of the menstrual cycle (the follicular phase).

Progesterone

Progesterone is another female sex hormone. It functions in the body to balance the effects of estrogen and is often referred to as the "relaxing hormone." Progesterone is produced after ovulation by the corpus luteum, a structure that forms in the ovary at the site of the follicle after release of the egg. This hormone dominates the second half of the menstrual cycle (**the luteal phase**). Progesterone's main job is to regulate the build-up of the uterine lining, helping to maintain the uterine lining if there is implantation/pregnancy. If there is no pregnancy, the progesterone levels decline, and the uterine lining is shed at the beginning the next menstrual cycle.

Menstrual Cycle

A menstrual cycle is measured by the number of days from the first day of one period to the first day of the next. Day 1 of the menstrual cycle is the first full bleeding day of the period. A typical cycle is approximately 24 to 35 days in length, with an average of 28 days for most women. It is not abnormal for a woman's cycle to occasionally vary in length.

On Day 1 of the menstrual cycle, estrogen and progesterone levels are low. Low levels of estrogen and progesterone signal the pituitary gland to produce FSH. The FSH begins the maturing process of an ovarian follicle.

The follicle produces more estrogen to prepare the uterus for pregnancy—primarily by prompting the development of the uterine lining. Sometime around Days 12 to 16, elevated estrogen levels trigger a sharp rise in LH secretion by the pituitary gland, causing ovulation—the release of the egg from the follicle.

The ruptured follicle, or corpus luteum, now secretes progesterone and estrogen to continue to prepare the uterus for pregnancy. If the egg is not fertilized, estrogen and progesterone levels drop, and on Day 28, you get your period.

The menstrual cycle occurs in three phases: follicular, ovulatory, and luteal. The first phase of the cycle is the follicular phase, and the third phase of the cycle is the luteal phase. Midway through the cycle, between Days 12 and 16, is the ovulatory phase, when ovulation occurs.

A woman is at the peak of her fertility from approximately three days before ovulation to one day after ovulation. Knowing your fertility window and understanding other aspects of your menstrual cycle are important for the following reasons:

1. Knowing your fertility window will allow you to time intercourse to your most fertile days.

2. The improper hormonal regulation of your menstrual cycle could be a reason why you aren't achieving your goal of becoming pregnant.

3. Understanding your menstrual cycle makes it easier to know which interventions are going to work best for you, depending on the exact nature of your hormonal imbalances.

4. Pathological conditions—such as polycystic ovarian syndrome (PCOS), endometriosis, and premenstrual

syndrome (PMS)—can be linked to an overabundance of estrogen compared to progesterone.

How Do You Monitor Your Menstrual Cycle?

Your body temperature dips slightly just before your ovary releases an egg. Then, 24 hours after the egg's release, your temperature rises and stays elevated for several days. Before ovulation, a woman's basal body temperature (BBT, the body temperature when fully at rest) averages between 36.1°C (97°F) and 36.4°C (97.5°F). After ovulation, it rises to a level between 36.4°C (97.6°F) and 37.0°C (98.6°F).

You can track your cycle by measuring your BBT every morning. Take your temperature at the same time every day before getting out of bed. Record the results on a chart or in a fertility app. If you have a generally regular cycle, the chart will help you predict when you will ovulate next. As your body senses the shifts that indicate the imminent release of an egg from the ovary, it begins to ready itself for the incoming sperm and to maximize the egg's chance of getting fertilized.

Important signs you can watch for include changes in the appearance, quantity, and consistency of cervical mucous. I have found that many women pay little attention to their cervical mucous. However, monitoring the mucus is an excellent way to understand your monthly cycle.

Once your period ends, it is typical to have little or no cervical discharges. When discharges begin again, they should be white in colour. As you get closer to ovulation, the discharges should increase in amount and become thinner and stretchy, similar in consistency to egg whites. These mucous characteristics, which usually start one to two days before the BBT increase, last between one and three days for most women. The mucous becomes thinner to aid the movement of sperm as they swim to reach the egg. If you notice this thinning, it is time to get busy in the bedroom.

Another way to monitor for ovulation at home involves the use of ovulation test strips. These strips measure your LH levels, showing a positive result when the levels rise to a certain point. The LH increases to allow the ovary to release an egg. With a typical 28-day cycle, you should start to use the strips around Day 10 and keep using them until you get a positive result. If you have a shorter cycle than 25 days, start using them earlier. The test strips can be expensive, so I strongly encourage women to monitor the other signs of ovulation and to use the strips only if they aren't seeing the other signs.

Returning to the BBT measurements, they should indicate, in healthy conditions, that the follicular phase lasts between 11 and 14 days. After ovulation, the luteal phase should also last between 11 and 14 days. If your follicular phase is shorter than 11 days, this can indicate that there is not enough time for the oocytes (immature eggs) to mature properly. If your follicular phase lasts from 12 to 20 days, there likely is enough time for proper oocyte development. If you are ovulating before Day 12, a botanical nutritional supplement called *Tribulus terrestris* (commonly called tribulus) could be helpful at lengthening the follicular phase. Speak to your health professional or naturopathic doctor about appropriate dosing.

During your luteal phase, once your temperature has increased, it should stay elevated for between 11 and 15 days. If the temperature does not remain elevated for at least 11 days, this can be an indicator that your progesterone level isn't staying elevated. To help keep progesterone levels up, it is important to implement some of the stress-reduction techniques discussed later in this book.

If you have already implemented stress reduction and are still seeing an abbreviated luteal phase, you can try a botanical called chaste tree (*Vitex agnus-castus*) to help support progesterone production[1]. Chaste tree usually requires about three cycles to produce a full effect. If you are under the care of a fertility specialist, you will likely be prescribed progesterone as a cream, suppository, or injection, resulting in an immediate increase in levels of the hormone. This is the approach taken in cases of IVF.

Imbalances of estrogen to progesterone can be detected through monitoring. Such imbalances may result in the following conditions[2]:

- Premenstrual syndrome (PMS)
- Polycystic ovarian syndrome (PCOS)
- Endometriosis
- Heavy menstrual flow
- Irregular cycle

Monitoring hormonal levels throughout the entire length of the cycle is important. This will tell you if your particular imbalance involves high estrogen levels and normal progesterone levels, or normal estrogen levels and low progesterone levels. There will be different treatment approaches depending on which condition applies to you.

In some cases, during monitoring, a woman may notice no increase in temperature and no obvious signs of ovulation. Such anovulation cycles are common in patients with PCOS. They can also occur due to other conditions, including a low percentage of body fat, high levels of prolactin (usually related to stress), and other hormonal imbalances. If anovulation is suspected, I would recommend seeking the care of a fertility clinic to get such tests as transvaginal ultrasound and hormonal monitoring blood work. These tests will help determine the reason for not ovulating.

Assignments

You should now have a basic understanding of hormonal functions and ovulation monitoring, including monitoring for cervical mucous, BBT, and LH level. To reinforce this understanding, take the time to complete the following assignments:

- Download a fertility app or obtain a BBT tracking chart (see example below).
- Monitor and record your body temperature first thing every morning.
- Record any observed changes in cervical mucous.
- Watch for positive results on LH strips (if you are not seeing changes with the other methods or as confirmation for the other methods).

In addition, keep track of the days on which you have intercourse. Ideally you will have intercourse at least twice per week throughout your cycle.

In the next chapter, we will begin to focus more sharply on how to optimize your fertility.

CHAPTER 3
BASICS OF SUPPLEMENTATION

IN THIS CHAPTER, we are going to discuss the basic supplements which I recommend be taken by all women and men to increase the chances of conception. We will cover the importance of prenatal vitamins, essential fatty acids, vitamin D, probiotics, and some antioxidants. Supplements can provide a significant benefit to women and men who are trying to conceive, but not all supplement manufacturers follow the same standards. Depending on where you live, there can be substantial differences in the quality, efficacy, and safety of the supplements you are taking. Preconception and pregnancy are crucial phases for the healthy development of your baby. Thus, it is paramount that you ensure the quality and integrity of what you are putting into your body.

At the end of this chapter, you will be able to:

- Identify the form of each nutrient you should look for on supplement labels

BASICS OF SUPPLEMENTATION

- Identify ingredients to avoid in your supplements
- List questions that you should ask your supplement provider

Issues to Consider

There are several issues to consider when choosing your supplements. These include the following:

1. In what format does the nutrient get delivered? It could be a capsule, tablet, liquid, powder, softgel or chewable. Tablets are the most difficult format for the body to break down into nutrients that can be properly absorbed. Tablets also contain a relatively large amount of fillers and binders, which may result in adverse effects in sensitive patients. Chewable and gummy products often contain many non-therapeutic ingredients. Additionally, with these products you often must take several doses compared to using capsules or liquids. Capsules, liquids, and powders usually have good absorption as well as fewer fillers and non-therapeutic ingredients.

2. Supplements should be free of potentially harmful ingredients, such as certain dyes. Examples of such dyes include FD&C Red No. 40 (aluminum lake), Yellow No. 6, Blue No. 1, talc, and shellac glaze. Some dyes have been found to be carcinogens (contribute to cancer growth) in animal studies so are best to be avoided when possible.

3. The supplement manufacturer should be able to prove the quality of the product. To do this, they should use a third-party laboratory to test each lot of their product and each raw material for purity, identity,

and lack of toxins or other contaminants. Speak to your prescribing health professional or pharmacist to confirm if the supplements you are using undergo this type of testing.

Prenatal Vitamins

Prenatal vitamin supplements are essential during the time you are trying to conceive, as well as when you know you are pregnant. However, all prenatals are not created equal. There are some great prenatals on the market, but also some of less desirable quality.

When choosing a prenatal, the various forms of the vitamins are important to consider. The following list displays the optimal forms and less desirable forms of several vitamin supplements.

Supplement	Optimal Forms	Less Desirable Forms
Calcium	Citrate or malate	Carbonate
Zinc	Citrate or picolinate	Oxide
Folate	Folate or L-5-MTHF (L-5-methyltetrahydrofolate)	Folic acid
B12	Methylcobalamin	Cyanocobalamin
Iron	Citrate or glycinate	Ferrous fumarate
Magnesium	Citrate, malate, or glycinate	Oxide

For folate supplements, you would ideally want the prenatal to contain either folate or L-5-methyltetrahydofolate (L-5-MTHF), rather than folic acid. Folic acid is a synthetic substance that is not as easily converted to its active form in the body. You have a gene that codes your ability to convert folate into its active form, L-5-MTHF. About 15 percent of the population have two copies of this gene, making them unable to convert folate to active L-5-MTHF. Approximately 50 percent of the population have a reduced ability to do this conversion sufficiently. If you have a limited ability to convert and are mainly consuming synthetic folic acid through prenatal supplements and fortified foods, you may face higher rates of miscarriage and embryonic neural tube defects, as well as such conditions as depression, attention-deficit/hyperactivity disorder, and autism for you and your baby[3]. For this reason, if I don't know the genetic status of a woman, I always recommend taking a supplement with the active form of folate, as well as limiting intake of synthetic folic acid through foods. Most of the grain products sold in North America are fortified with synthetic folic acid. An excellent natural source of folate is green leafy vegetables.

In general, you want to see higher levels of B vitamins in your prenatal supplements, as they will aid with energy production. You also want to ensure that the dose of your prenatal is between two and four capsules per day. A once-a-day dose will not be enough to provide the essential nutrients that you require during the preconception phase.

In terms of a multivitamin, you want to ensure that you are getting at minimum, B12, active folate (5-MTHFR), zinc, and vitamin E (with tocopherols and selenium). Some antioxidants and amino acids are also potentially useful. This vitamin information can be applied to the male partner as well as the female.

For a man, the preconception phase is important for making healthy sperm and deficiency of any of these nutrients can have a negative impact on sperm health. We will discuss this subject further in chapter 13 Optimizing sperm health.

Probiotics

Probiotics are beneficial bacteria that are necessary to support digestion and immune function. These microbes enhance your ability to properly absorb nutrients, and they help keep your immune system in balance. Balanced immune function is essential during preconception, as an imbalanced immune system can impair the fertility of some women. This includes women who have autoimmune conditions, such as Hashimoto's thyroiditis, celiac disease or rheumatoid arthritis, and women with such conditions as allergies or asthma.

There is a wealth of research showing that numerous strains of probiotic bacteria can have a beneficial impact on the immune system. Certain strains help shift how the immune system functions and responds to different bacterial or viral exposures. For example, *Lactobacillus rhamnosus* has been shown to produce immune-balancing effects. This microbe should be one of the strains in your probiotic—especially if you have an autoimmune condition, allergies/asthma, or eczema[4].

The following guidelines are useful in choosing a probiotic:

1. You want the probiotic product to be multi-strain. This means that it should contain more than just a single strain of bacteria. Between 8 and 15 strains is optimal.

2. The probiotic should contain a combination of several strains of *Lactobacillus* and *Bifidobacterium*.

3. The total dose per capsule for a healthy person is approximately 10 billion cultures per capsule. If the probiotic is taken after antibiotic use, it is usually preferable to take 50 to 100 billion cultures per capsule for 30 to 90 days.

4. Ideally, the product should have an enteric coating or be pH-activated. The reason for this is that stomach acid can kill both harmful and helpful strains of

bacteria. A probiotic capsule that doesn't dissolve in the low pH of the stomach is preferable to ensure that the maximum number of probiotics reach your small intestine, where they become active.

5. The bacterial cultures of probiotics should remain alive and viable during storage. It is best to choose a probiotic that is kept refrigerated, as this will keep the bacteria alive longer to ensure their beneficial effects. If you are choosing a shelf-stable or non-refrigerated probiotic, you should try to find out if the manufacturer conducted stability testing to ensure that the bacteria can survive at higher temperatures for prolonged periods.

Essential Fatty Acids

Essential fatty acids are fats that we must consume in our diets because our bodies don't have the ability to make them. Their designation as "essential" fatty acids means that we cannot survive without them. Both omega-3 and omega-6 fatty acids are considered essential. In the typical North American diet, we generally consume an adequate amount of omega-6 fatty acids but an inadequate amount of omega-3 fatty acids.

In men, optimal omega-3 levels have been shown to improve sperm production and increase the chances of successful conception. In women, omega-3 fatty acids help to regulate hormones, increase blood flow to the uterus (important for uterine lining thickness), and increase ovulatory cervical mucus (needed to help the sperm reach the egg).

There are three types of omega-3 fatty acids—alpha-linolenic acid (ALA), eicosapentaenoic acid (EPA), and docosahexaenoic acid (DHA). Your body has the ability to convert ALA into EPA and then DHA, but the conversion rate for most people is very low[5]. Considering this limitation, the best dietary source of omega-3 fatty acids is fish, which contains EPA and DHA.

When choosing a fish-oil supplement, it is essential to know the quality of the oil, including whether it has been tested for potential contaminants. Possible contaminants include toxic metals, such as mercury and lead, and other pollutants, such as dioxins and polychlorinated biphenyls (PCBs). These pollutants can contaminate our water supplies, and they become increasingly concentrated as they move up the food chain. It is imperative that manufacturers of fish oils molecularly distill the oils and test them for any impurities. Please confirm with your prescribing health professional or pharmacist that the manufacturer can provide independent test results showing the quality of its oil. If the company is unable to provide such test results, I would avoid using its products. This information is especially important for any products that might contain toxic metals, as these substances will pass directly through the placenta to the baby. This could include omega 3 fatty acids, any herbs grown in soils that could have exposure to toxic chemicals or pesticides, as well as nutrients sourced from animals who have been fed on non-organic foods.

Regarding dosing of essential fatty acids, you want to get between 1 and 2 grams of combined EPA/DHA per day. In capsule form, this will amount to between one and four capsules. In high-potency liquid form, it will be between 1 teaspoon- 1 tablespoon.

Vitamin D

Sunlight produces a vital nutrient for us by triggering a cascade of chemical reactions within the body. When your skin and eyes are directly exposed to sunlight, the light prompts your body to manufacture vitamin D. Without sunlight to produce vitamin D, you can suffer from bone loss, depression, sleep disorders, immune deficiencies, and hormonal imbalances.

Vitamin D has properties of both a vitamin and a hormone. The vitamin is essential for bone development, hormone production, a healthy nervous system, and balanced neurotransmitter levels. It is responsible for the absorption and utilization of calcium, the most abundant mineral in the body. Without vitamin D3, our cells cannot use calcium effectively.

A simple blood test can assess the status of vitamin D in the body. Details of this test and other laboratory testing will be discussed in a later chapter. At this point, we can note that many people in Canada and other countries in the northern latitudes use supplements to ensure they have adequate vitamin D levels during the winter months. It is generally recommended to use a supplement of at least 2,000 international units (IUs) of vitamin D3 per day.

There is research showing that women who are vitamin-D deficient have a more challenging time conceiving and maintaining pregnancy[6]. There are also several studies that have linked low vitamin D to conditions that can make both achieving and maintaining a pregnancy more challenging such as Hashimoto's and PCOS[7]. I have had patients who unsuccessfully tried IVF procedures, and once their vitamin D levels were corrected, they were able to conceive naturally.

Antioxidants

Coenzyme Q10 (CoQ10) is an enzyme made in the liver that functions as an antioxidant. It supports the functioning of mitochondria. Mitochondria are the energy power house of your cells and are responsible for producing energy in your cells. Properly functioning mitochondria are important for the quality of both sperm and egg cells. After the age of 30, mitochondrial function begins to decline. This is especially relevant to fertility, because your oocytes (immature eggs) have a high quantity of mitochondria, which produce the energy that aids in the maturation of the eggs. In a study of oocyte quality, researchers explored the link between impaired mitochondrial performance and oocyte deficits. They concluded that impaired mitochondrial performance caused by less-than-optimal CoQ10 availability can lead to infertility in older women[8] . A general recommendation for both women and men over age 30 is to take 100 milligrams (mg) of CoQ10 twice per day to enhance fertility.

An important amino acid called L-carnitine works alongside CoQ10 to enable CoQ10 to enter your cells. If you are deficient in L-carnitine, even CoQ10 supplements may be unable to allow your cells to achieve sufficient energy production[9]. L-carnitine can be obtained only from animal sources of protein. Thus, if you are vegetarian or vegan, you are likely deficient in this amino acid. If you have any concerns about conditions such as fibromyalgia, chronic fatigue, or poor egg quality, I would suggest adding at least 1 gram (g) of L-carnitine into your daily regimen.

The supplements discussed in this chapter will provide your body with an improved base level of health and ensure that basic deficiencies are avoided. There are several additional supplements that may be helpful, depending on your individual situation.

Assignments

- Check the ingredients in your prenatal supplement. If the ingredients do not include the substances described in this chapter, consider purchasing a replacement product.
- If you are not currently eating fish at least twice a week, consider adding an omega-3 fatty acid supplement to your diet.

BASICS OF SUPPLEMENTATION

- Get your vitamin-D level assessed to see if you need to take a supplement.

- If you are over age 30, consider adding an antioxidant supplement, such as CoQ10 and L-carnitine.

- If you have any immune or digestive concerns, look at supplementation with a probiotic.

- If you have more questions about supplements speak to your Naturopathic doctor and/or visit Enhance Fertility https://enhancefertility.ca/ for products and further education.

CHAPTER 4
SCREENING LABS

RESULTS OF CERTAIN laboratory tests, referred to as screening labs, allow you to understand your baseline health. This is important knowledge to have before trying to get pregnant. Depending on where you are in your fertility journey, this lab work may or may not have been done already. If you are currently under the care of a fertility specialist, it is likely that the majority of these tests have been completed. I strongly recommend that you keep copies of your laboratory reports for your records. You should know what blood work has been run, and you should keep your results in the optimal ranges. This chapter covers those lab tests that are especially relevant to fertility and pregnancy.

By the end of this chapter, you will be able to:

- Name the screening labs that are most important
- Identify the optimal values of these labs

SCREENING LABS

- Feel confident speaking to your doctor about these labs

Preconception Screening Labs

Below is a list of screening labs that should be performed during the preconception period.

- Anti-Mullerian hormone (AMH)—if considering IVF
- Cholesterol panel
- Complete blood count (CBC)
- Estradiol
- Fasting blood sugar and hemoglobin A1c (HbA1c)
- Ferritin
- Follicle-stimulating hormone (FSH)
- Homocysteine
- Liver and kidney chemistry
- Luteinizing hormone (LH)
- Progesterone (between Days 19-22)
- Prolactin
- Red blood cell- (RBC-) folate or serum/plasma folate (there are 2 different ways to assess folate levels so having one or the other done is sufficient)
- Sexually transmitted infections (STI)—chlamydia, gonorrhea, syphilis, HIV, hepatitis B and C
- Testosterone

- Thyroid panel- Including thyroid-stimulating hormone (TSH)/free thyroxine (T4)/free triiodothyronine (T3), TPO and anti-TG antibodies
- Vitamin B12
- Vitamin D

Compare the lab tests in this list to the blood work that you have already had done. If there are tests that haven't been completed, speak to your doctor or fertility specialist about having them run. For most tests, as long as the values come back within the stated reference range, you have nothing to be concerned about in that area. In the following text, I am going to focus on the tests that are at times overlooked, or that have reference ranges too wide for optimal health.

Let's start with nutrient screening. There are five main vitamin or mineral tests that should be run: vitamin B12, folate, homocysteine, ferritin, and vitamin D. Deficiencies in vitamin B12, folate, ferritin, or vitamin D—or elevated levels of homocysteine—can be contributing factors to infertility. In some cases, abnormal levels of these substances may lead to miscarriage.

Vitamin B12

Vitamin B12 is a water-soluble nutrient obtained in the diet mainly through meat, dairy products, eggs, and fish. If you are vegan or vegetarian and not taking a supplement, your B12 levels are likely low. Signs and symptoms of low B12 include the following:

- Fatigue
- Problems with mental focus and concentration
- Tinnitus

- Nerve pain or damage
- Anxiety
- Poor sleep
- Recurrent miscarriage
- Infertility
- High homocysteine levels
- Anemia

The reference range for vitamin B12 is between 153 and 655 picomoles per litre (pmol/L). I find that most women will feel better with a B12 level above 450 pmol/L. There are some patients who feel best being well above the top end of the range, so this is very individual for each person. If your lab value is below the reference range, B12 injections or B12 supplements (in hydroxocobalamin or methylcobalamin form) are essential for conception—and important to continue during pregnancy[10]. Some patients don't absorb B12 when taken orally, so using injections or sublingual options can achieve better results in these cases.

There are associations between low B12 status in the mother and increased rates of neurological problems in the baby, including autism, ADHD, and generalized anxiety. B12 deficiency can also have a major impact on sperm health[11]. Thus, it is important for the male partner to have his B12 level assessed.

Folate

Folate, or vitamin B9, has several of the same functions as B12. These vitamins can mask deficiencies of one another, so levels of both should be checked in preconception blood work. Low folate levels can lead to infertility, miscarriage, and neural tube defects in infants.

Folate levels can be assessed in two types of tests—one involving analysis of red blood cells (RBC) and the other involving analysis of blood serum or plasma. Assessed via RBC, the reference range for folate is greater than 630 nanomoles per litre (nmol/L). Assessed via plasma, the range is 4.5 to 45.3 nmol/L.

A good prenatal supplement should prevent deficiency of both B12 and folate. Nevertheless, analysis of the levels of these nutrients is necessary to ensure that your body is absorbing them efficiently.

Homocysteine

Homocysteine is not a nutrient in our diet. Rather, it is an amino acid that is synthesized in a process called methylation. This is a complex process, involving multiple nutrients, that is one of the most important detoxification pathways in the body. Proper functioning of methylation pathways is necessary to produce homocysteine at healthy levels.

Several studies have linked high homocysteine levels to heart disease, stroke, cancer, and autoimmune diseases, as well as infertility and early miscarriage[12]. The upper limit for homocysteine has yet to be clearly established. On most lab reports, the range is given as 5 to 15 micromoles per litre (μmol/L). However, some reports suggest that any reading over 6.8 μmol/L could be problematic.

Homocysteine can become elevated because of poor diet or high caffeine or alcohol intake. Vegetarians and vegans are at greater risk of elevated homocysteine because they tend to lack sufficient amounts of the nutrients needed for methylation, including folate, vitamins B6 and B12, and trimethyl glycine. There are also genetic factors that can leave you more prone to a high homocysteine reading.

If your homocysteine level is elevated but your folate or B12 levels are low, you need to increase your doses of B12 and folate/L-5-MTHF, and you should ensure that your prenatal supplement has some of the active form of B6 called pyridoxine (or pyridoxal) 5-phosphate. After taking this combination for six weeks, repeat your lab work to ensure that the homocysteine value has decreased.

Ferritin

Ferritin is your storage form of iron. As ferritin levels become depleted, you may experience fatigue, poor concentration, and problems with recovery after exercise. If your stores of ferritin are too low, your body won't be able to maintain a healthy pregnancy[13]. Test results for ferritin tend to be low if you have a heavy period, if you are a female athlete, or if you are vegetarian or vegan.

The reference range for ferritin in women is about 11 to 247 micrograms per litre (μg/L). (For men, the range is up to 300 μg/L.) In my practice, I will recommend supplements for any woman who has a ferritin reading under 50 μg/L, as I find that levels below that value can be problematic. Depending on the reading, your prenatal supplement may be enough to bring the level up. However, if your level is less than 20 μg/L, recommendations call for an additional iron supplement—either a heme source or an iron glycinate source. The iron supplement will help to ensure optimal ferritin absorption. It is also a great idea to focus your diet on iron-rich foods.

Vitamin D

The value of vitamin D supplements was discussed in the chapter on supplements. As previously noted, deficiency in vitamin D is especially prevalent in women with polycystic ovarian syndrome (PCOS) and such autoimmune disorders as Hashimoto's thyroiditis and rheumatoid arthritis[14]. A deficiency will impact your body's ability to synthesize the hormones that are essential for fertility purposes. In a study of women with anovulatory infertility, 93 percent of the women were found to be deficient in vitamin D. Supplementing to achieve optimal levels can help restore normal ovulatory function.

The reference range for vitamin D is 75 to 150 pmol/L. If your level is below this range, a vitamin D supplement of between 2,000 and 5,000 IU/day is usually needed. Always make sure that you take your vitamin D supplement with a dietary fat source to aid in the proper absorption of the vitamin.

Hormonal Health

When you are referred to a fertility clinic—before any treatment can be started—your specialist will usually recommend a series of lab tests and ultrasound scans during your cycle to develop an understanding about your cycle characteristics. Thus, if you are currently under the care of a fertility specialist, it is likely that tests of your female hormones have been run multiple times as part of your initial cycle monitoring.

If you are not under the care of a fertility specialist, blood work during the luteal phase, between Days 19 and 22, will determine if you have any problems with progesterone levels. Low progesterone is a common cause of early miscarriage, so it is important to know your status.

Levels of LH and FSH both surge around the time of ovulation. It is ideal to assess these levels, along with that of estradiol, around Day 3 if you have a regular menstrual cycle. Your testosterone and prolactin may be checked at the same time as the LH and FSH or at the time of progesterone assessment. If you need a refresher on these hormones, please refer to the previous discussion in the chapter 2 Hormonal Health.

Thyroid Function

There are three markers that are used to assess thyroid function—thyroid-stimulating hormone (TSH), free thyroxine (T4), and free triiodothyronine (T3). TSH is a hormone that comes from the pituitary gland. It prompts the thyroid gland to make T4, which travels through circulation to the tissues and is converted to the active thyroid hormone, T3. The reference range for TSH is usually given as 0.32 to 4.00 μg/L. However, many fertility specialists believe that this range is too wide and that the ideal TSH level should be below 2.5 μg/L.

It is important to run tests for all three thyroid markers, because some women will have normal TSH and T4 but low T3. Low levels of T3 will generally lead to symptoms associated with hypothyroidism, including weight gain, cold intolerance, dry/cracked heels, constipation, and fatigue. Thyroid problems tend to be underdiagnosed, but they are important to detect because thyroid malfunction can be a contributing factor to infertility.

High cortisol levels due to stress will impair your body's ability to convert T4 into T3. About 20 percent of the conversion of T4 to T3 occurs in the gastrointestinal tract. Thus, ensuring proper bacterial balance in the gut and proper digestive function will assist in optimizing conversion. The cofactors required for this conversion are selenium, zinc, copper, iodine, and L-tyrosine. A low T3 level can usually be corrected by taking a supplement containing these cofactors.

In some cases, a prescription thyroid hormone will be necessary to optimize thyroid function and improve symptoms of hypothyroidism. This hormone can be prescribed by your family doctor, your fertility specialist or by your naturopathic doctor.

Hashimoto's thyroiditis is an underdiagnosed autoimmune condition that often affects fertility. This condition can be indicated by tests for thyroid peroxidase (TPO) antibodies and thyroglobulin (TG) antibodies. These antibodies should be screened at the same time as the rest of the thyroid markers. Often patients that have low thyroid function actually have Hashimoto's thyroiditis. Elevated antibodies indicate this autoimmune condition which can have a direct impact on your ability to achieve as well as maintain a healthy pregnancy[15].

Anti-Mullerian Hormone

Assessment of anti-Mullerian hormone (AMH) does not have to be performed as part of a basic screen, but it does become relevant for patients considering IVF. AMH is secreted by the granulosa cells within the ovarian follicles. The blood level of this hormone is thought to reflect the size of the remaining egg supply within the ovaries. I have found that many women who have low AMH readings will become anxious or overly concerned about this test result. However, it is important to keep in mind that your AMH level does not reflect the active maturation or quality of your eggs.

Women with PCOS produce many small follicles and often have a high level of AMH; whereas, women closer to menopause usually have a low AMH. Generally speaking, women with higher AMH readings have better response to IVF treatment because they will usually have more eggs retrieved. But a low AMH reading does not necessarily mean that you won't be able to conceive or that an IVF cycle won't work for you. A study led by fertility specialist Richard Sherbahn, MD, determined that low AMH levels in women under age 35 were not correlated with poor IVF outcomes.

The test for AMH is relatively new, so its reference ranges are still being debated among fertility doctors. I encourage my patients to not be discouraged by this testing. If your AMH is high, it is likely that you could be hyper stimulated with medication in your IVF cycle. This is something that your fertility specialist will discuss with you.

Summary

You can achieve a base level of health and proper functioning to benefit your fertility by completing the lab work that is recommended in this chapter and by addressing any imbalances. This approach will ensure that nutrient depletion or hormonal imbalances are not causing or contributing to your infertility or recurrent miscarriages. Improving these values will also help you to boost your energy, sharpen your mental clarity, and optimize your overall health.

Assignments

- Refer to the list of lab screening tests previously presented and check the listed tests against the lab work that you have already had.

- Ask your healthcare provider for a copy of all your blood work if you do not already have a copy. Note any differences between the list in this chapter and the tests that you have had. If any tests have not been done, ask your healthcare provider about them.

CHAPTER 5
THE IMPACT OF STRESS AND THE IMPORTANCE OF EXERCISE

IT IS COMMONLY known that psychological stress is likely to impact a woman's ability to conceive and maintain a healthy pregnancy. But what exactly is stress and how does it play such an important role in not only fertility and pregnancy, but also in overall health?

In this chapter, you will learn three important concepts:

1. The physical and emotional impact of stress
2. Determining how well your body is coping with stressors
3. Implementing techniques to better manage your stress

THE IMPACT OF STRESS AND THE IMPORTANCE OF EXERCISE

Stress Prevalence

Stress is a normal part of everyday life, and it is what allows us to have productive days. When the body is under perceived stress, your adrenal glands secrete a hormone called cortisol. Cortisol contributes to a natural rhythm in the body, helping you to wake in the morning and sleep at night. In addition, if you are in a life-threatening situation, your body should respond by secreting cortisol and preparing for the "fight or flight" response. However, in modern Western society, the body and mind are under chronic stress, causing the natural rhythm to get out of sync and leading to either an overproduction or underproduction of cortisol.

High stress is extremely common today. In a large study conducted in 2017 by the American Psychological Association called *Stress in America*, women aged 18 to 55 reported an average stress level of 5.1 on a scale of 1 to 10 (with 10 being the highest stress level)[16]. That was 2 points higher than what is considered healthy. About 23 percent of the surveyed women reported experiencing extreme daily stress, at levels of 8 to 10. The women acknowledged the importance of stress management, but few felt they were doing a good job of it.

Women who are struggling with their fertility generally fall within the group experiencing daily stress levels between 8 and 10. I find in practice that some women fully acknowledge the effects of stress in their lives, while others downplay its implications. Even if you don't feel that you are stressed, implementing the following techniques will have a major positive impact on your daily life.

When stress becomes a chronic problem, it can have a negative impact on the health of your oocytes, your eggs, and your future babies. Thus, you need to become aware of the symptoms of stress. These symptoms include the following:

- Headaches

- Anxiety
- Irritability
- Low energy (such as generalized fatigue throughout the day or a mid-afternoon dip in energy)
- Poor digestion (such as constipation or irritable bowel syndrome)
- Premenstrual syndrome
- Short, long, or irregular menstrual cycle
- Heavy periods
- Poor sleep quality (such as a pattern of waking between 3 am and 5 am)

When my stress levels become chronically elevated, the first physical change I notice is in my menstrual cycle, which shortens from 28 to 22 days. In addition, I have stronger PMS symptoms, I become extremely irritable, and I have limited patience for my loved ones.

Abnormal Cortisol Levels

One of the ways in which high stress can impact pregnancy is through a process called "progesterone steal". Progesterone is a precursor hormone for cortisol, a steroid hormone produced by the adrenal glands. Generally, the more cortisol your body needs to make, the less progesterone it has in reserve. If a woman has low progesterone levels, her body cannot maintain a pregnancy because either there is isn't enough time for implantation before progesterone drops, or an early miscarriage can occur.

The high cortisol levels resulting from stress can promote inflammation in the body. Certain conditions, such as PCOS or endometriosis, can be exacerbated by higher cortisol levels. For a patient with PCOS, the higher cortisol could lead to anovulation. With endometriosis, the endometrial tissue could become increasingly engorged, leading to more pain and further abnormal tissue growth.

Elevated cortisol levels can also lead to elevations of another hormone, called prolactin. Prolactin is normally elevated only in women who are breast-feeding. Abnormal increases in prolactin block or impair the activity of hormones that help with egg development and ovulation. This can be a reason why a woman isn't ovulating regularly.

There are tests to determine if your adrenals are responding in a healthy way to stress and if you are regulating your cortisol levels properly. One such test measures orthostatic blood pressure. With this test, you first lay down and relax for two minutes. You then take your blood pressure, stand up, and take it again. If your adrenals are functioning properly, you should see the top blood-pressure number, or systolic blood pressure, increase by about 10 points between the two readings. If you do not see this change, it may be a sign that your adrenal glands could benefit from nutritional or herbal based support such as ashwagandha and holy basil.

Another test of adrenal function is called the Koenisberg test. This is a urine-based test that can be performed in the office of your naturopathic doctor. The test provides a general idea of how your body is responding to stress by examining the amount of salt in the urine. Salt-water balance is a function of the adrenal glands. Yet another test of adrenal function is the four-point salivary cortisol test, in which cortisol secretion is monitored at different points throughout the day. The results provide a good indication of how your body is responding to stress during the day, including whether you are oversecreting or under-secreting cortisol.

Regulating Cortisol

A number of strategies are available to help regulate your cortisol level and its impact on your body. I have found the three strategies discussed here to be highly effective.

1. **Exercise.** For most of my patients—and for myself—exercise has been shown to be a major stress reliever. Unfortunately, exercise is often the first thing that drops out of a daily schedule when a person gets busy. It should be the last.

   Exercising for up to 60 minutes a day will help lower your cortisol levels. The exercise does not need to be of high intensity. It could be walking, yoga, swimming, weight training, dancing—anything that gets your body moving and that you enjoy. If you can keep your body moving for even 20 minutes every day, this will have a significant impact on your cortisol regulation. However, if you do enjoy high-intensity exercise, such exercises as high-intensity interval training (HIIT) and Tabata-style training can lead to increases in growth hormone. This, in turn, can lead to improvements in regulation of cortisol and various other hormones.

   It is important to keep in mind that whatever exercise routine you choose should not add extra stress into your life. For example, if you must race across town after leaving work early to fight traffic to get to your yoga class, this is not the best choice for you. It would be better to choose a yoga video and do it at home or find a studio that is close to work or home.

2. **A consistent schedule.** Your body thrives on routine. For your hormones to work most effectively, you should go to bed and get up at the same time every day. If possible, you should also exercise and eat around the

same time each day. When your body "knows" consistently what to expect, the adrenal glands can start to cycle cortisol properly again. I understand that a consistent schedule may not be possible for everyone. Nevertheless, the more consistent you can be, the easier it will be for your body to make appropriate hormonal adjustments. You may find any consistency extremely difficult to achieve if your job involves shift work with rotating days and nights or frequent travel in different time zones. If this is the case for you, I am not suggesting that you quit your job. Rather, I urge you to do your best to regularly implement other stress-reducing techniques.

3. **Diaphragm breathing or yoga breathing.** When you engage the diaphragm for breathing, this muscle between your stomach and lungs takes your nervous system from its stressed mode to its relaxed mode. To engage your diaphragm, these four steps should be followed:

> Step 1: Sit comfortably with your feet planted on the ground.
>
> Step 2: Place one hand over your chest and the other hand over your stomach.
>
> Step 3: Inhale deeply through your nose so that you feel the hand over your stomach move up, and then down as you exhale.
>
> Step 4: Repeat this process at least 10 times.

If you go to yoga classes your instructors are trained to teach proper breathing techniques. These are also effective at engaging your diaphragm in breathing. If you have never done breathing exercises, it may be difficult to remember to do them. Having something to cue you throughout the day is helpful. For example, you could take 10 deep breaths before each meal and before each bedtime. This would ensure that you check your breathing at least four times per day. Some women will find it helpful to focus on their breathing whenever they are feeling stressed or irritable in order to help them move out of that frame of mind. You can do breathing exercises anytime and anywhere, so there is no excuse for not implementing them into your daily regimen.

If these three strategies are not enough to restore adrenal function, there are also supplements and herbs that could be helpful. In particular, vitamin B5 and herbs called adaptogens (such as holy basil, ginseng, and licorice) can help to restore the healthy function of the adrenal system. For more advice regarding supplementation and cortisol regulation, you should consult your naturopathic doctor.

Assignments

- Consciously try to maintain as consistent a schedule as possible, going to sleep and getting up at the same time each day, and exercising and eating meals around the same time daily.

- Start doing yoga exercises or diaphragm breathing, spending at least a couple minutes before each meal focused on your breath. This will go a long way toward helping your body maintain natural cortisol rhythm.

- Record notes on how a more consistent schedule and breathing exercises affect your sleep pattern, energy level, overall mood and sense of well-being, and menstrual cycle.

CHAPTER 6
THE IMPORTANCE OF SLEEP

SLEEP HAS A major impact on both your mental health and physical health, and it substantially affects your daily functioning. Chemicals in the body called neurotransmitters help to control our sleeping and waking times by acting on different nerve cells in the brain.

In this chapter, you will learn the following:

- How sleep impacts your hormonal regulation and immune function
- Strategies for improving your sleep quality

Stages of Sleep

There are five stages of sleep—stages 1, 2, 3, 4, and REM (rapid eye movement). The first four stages progress to REM sleep and then continue to cycle multiple times per night, with each cycle lasting between 90 and 110 minutes.

Stage-1 sleep is a light sleep from which you can easily drift in and out of. Entering stage 2, brain wave activity starts to slow down, and eye movements stop. As you progress to stage 3, the slower and longer delta brain waves begin, but they are interspersed with shorter, faster waves. By stage 4, the brain produces delta waves almost exclusively. Stage 3 and stage 4 are both considered deep sleep, when there is no eye movement or muscle activity. When you transition into REM sleep, breathing becomes more rapid, skeletal muscles become temporarily paralyzed but eye movement increases, and dreaming can occur.

Going through your sleep cycles allows your body and mind to heal and repair. This is also the time when your immune system is functioning at its best. Your hormones go through cycles based on your sleep patterns, so good-quality sleep aids in the regulation of your menstrual cycle. In addition, sleep is crucial to your body's ability to regulate cortisol.

Cortisol and Sleep

We discussed the role of cortisol in the previous chapter, but as a reminder, this is a hormone produced by your adrenal glands, associated with stress, and it can affect fertility. The natural rhythm of cortisol is to increase in the morning to help you wake up, to drop throughout the day, and to reach its lowest level in the late evening, allowing you to fall asleep. When we are under a great deal of stress, cortisol secretion from the adrenal glands increases. Continued secretion can, over time, have a negative impact on your menstrual cycle and your chance of conception. The more cortisol your body produces, the less progesterone you will have. This is the previously noted process called "progesterone steal".

THE IMPORTANCE OF SLEEP

A master hormone called pregnenolone can function in several ways, including serving to produce estrogen and to produce progesterone. The progesterone can then be converted to cortisol. If your body needs to make too much cortisol in response to stress or other factors, you may be left deficient in progesterone. Progesterone is your predominant hormone during the luteal phase (the second half of the menstrual cycle), and it is essential for the embryo to be implanted in the uterus. Furthermore, the proper balance of your estrogen to progesterone is relevant for conditions such as fibrocystic breast disease, endometriosis, and PCOS. Good-quality sleep is important for all these processes and conditions.

Evaluating Your Sleep

How do you know if you're getting enough sleep? Ideally, sleep should range from 6.5 to 9 hours each night. One way to tell if your sleep is sufficient is based on how you feel in the morning. If you are someone who wakes up feeling groggy and likes to hit the snooze button multiple times, you are likely not getting enough sleep. If you can wake up on your own without the use of an alarm clock and feel rested, that is a good indication you are getting enough sleep. Another way to evaluate your sleep is based on your energy level throughout the day. Are you someone who could fall asleep at any point in the day if you aren't keeping busy? Or do you usually feel like you have good energy to get through the day? I often see patients who tell me they have good energy only when they are keeping busy or using stimulants, such as caffeine. I usually advise these individuals to try to get more sleep.

Many of us lead extremely busy and hectic lives, and we don't stop and check in with ourselves about how we are feeling. You need to occasionally take the time to stop and monitor yourself. When you do, if you feel completely exhausted, that is a strong indicator that you aren't getting sufficient sleep.

In any given day, you should not need to rely on caffeinated beverages, such as coffee, tea, energy drinks, or cola products for energy. If you do, your sleep is likely insufficient. If you experience midafternoon energy drops, this could also be an indicator of lack of sleep, leading to cortisol dysregulation.

Improving Your Sleep Quality

I realize that this sounds simplistic, but the first step toward ensuring high-quality sleep is going to bed when you start to feel tired. When you begin feeling tired, instead of turning on the TV or continuing to push through to get your work done, go to bed. It is often the case that not listening to your body's fatigue cues will cause you to become overtired. This can result in you having greater difficulty falling asleep when you do go to bed. Another behavior you want to avoid is falling asleep on the couch or other non-bed locations, and then waking up to go to bed. This habit will disrupt your sleep cycle and hormone regulation.

To be able to properly regulate sleep, you need to optimize your body's ability to make a hormone called melatonin. Your body normally starts to secrete melatonin around bedtime, making you feel sleepy. It continues to be secreted throughout the night to help you remain asleep. To maximize your melatonin production, you need to have complete darkness in your sleep environment. This means no nightlight, no lights on the alarm clock, no light coming through the windows, and no other kind of light. A common cause of low melatonin production is using backlit electronic products—such as cell phones, tablets, or computers—just before going to bed. It is best to stop using all such products ideally 2 hours before bed. If this isn't possible for you, there are glasses you can use that block up to 95% of the blue light emitted from screens that will protect your melatonin production.

THE IMPORTANCE OF SLEEP

If you are having difficulty falling asleep or if you wake up frequently during the night, this will obviously disrupt your hormone production. There are natural sleep aids that can help. For example, a supplement containing melatonin can be helpful in inducing sleep. You may also try drinking a calming tea (non-caffeinated) before bedtime to help the nervous system relax. This kind of tea contains such herbal ingredients as passionflower, chamomile, and lavender. Certain other substances—such as gamma-aminobutyric acid (GABA), L-theanine, and lavender essential oil—can aid later stages of sleep to improve the chances of getting a full-night sleep.

Low levels of progesterone can also impact your sleep cycle. This may be the reason that you find your sleep being disrupted in the week before your period. The best way to check your progesterone level is to ask your health practitioner to perform a blood test or a salivary hormone panel during the luteal phase, or second half, of your menstrual cycle. Ideally, you would have your blood drawn between Days 19 and 22 (reminder: Day 1 is the first day of you period). Alternatively, you could have a salivary hormone test during this same window. If you have an irregular menstrual cycle, it could be helpful to have a month-long salivary assessment, in which a salivary sample is analyzed every three days through your entire menstrual cycle. This form of testing would also be useful for women who have such conditions as endometriosis or PCOS, in which hormones are imbalanced. In these cases, supporting your adrenal system to help regulate your cortisol is essential. Your healthcare provider can advise you in this regard. If the reason for your low progesterone is stress, implementing the techniques discussed in the previous chapter will be helpful.

If your progesterone remains low, you might consider using an herb called chaste tree. Chaste tree helps your body increase production of both progesterone and LH, thereby improving hormonal regulation. If you find that none of these steps restore your hormonal balance, you can discuss prescription progesterone with your health professional. There are several options for progesterone-containing prescription products. These include bio-identical creams, vaginal suppositories, and oral or injectable medications that are used during the luteal phase of your menstrual cycle.

Assignments

Your sleep-wake patterns have a direct impact on your body's hormone regulation and your ability to conceive and maintain a pregnancy. To improve your sleep-wake patterns, try incorporating these behaviors into your daily routine:

- Make a habit of going to bed when you first notice you are feeling tired.

- Do not use any backlit electronic products for 2 hours before going to bed or use protective eye wear.

- When you go to bed, make sure that your room is completely dark.

- If you still aren't sleeping well speak to your health care professional

CHAPTER 7
ARE EATING ORGANIC AND NON-GMO FOODS IMPORTANT?

DO YOU NEED to consume organic foods to improve your fertility? If so, do all your foods need to be organic or only some? This chapter speaks about the importance and relevance to fertility of organic foods and foods that are not made with genetically modified organisms (GMO). Also discussed are the types of fish that are best to include in your diet.

By the end of the chapter, you should have a good understanding of:

- Fruits and vegetables that should ideally be eaten as organic, as well as those that are acceptable to eat as non-organic

- Reasons why the amount of GMO foods in your diet should be minimized
- Fish that are best to include in your diet, including those with the lowest amount of toxicity

Organic Foods

What exactly is an organic food? Each country has different guidelines for labelling organic foods. This section specifically describes the guidelines in Canada. Guidelines in the United States are similar.

For a farm to be certified organic in Canada, it must demonstrate that it uses management practices that seek to nurture ecosystems to achieve sustainable productivity. Certain chemical substances and techniques are not allowed during the cultivation or handling processes. Products must be free of genetic engineering. Synthetic pesticides cannot be used. Fertilizers cannot contain any banned substances. Containers in storage cannot contain synthetic fungicides. The raising of farm animals cannot involve synthetic antibiotics or parasiticides, and animals cannot be fed diets that include GMO products. These are the main points, but there are many additional criteria for organic status.

Therefore, if a food product has the Canadian Food Inspection Agency (CFIA) organic label or, similarly, the United States Department of Agriculture (USDA) organic label, you can be confident that it hasn't been sprayed with synthetic chemicals and that it is GMO-free.

It has been well-documented that foods farmed and grown organically have higher levels of vitamins and nutrients than their nonorganic counterparts. Furthermore, they also taste better. Fruits and vegetables that are organically grown are allowed to ripen in their natural environment in a natural length of time, maximizing the development of antioxidants.

By contrast, the majority of nonorganic produce is picked before it is ripe and before antioxidants have developed sufficiently. Chemicals are used to make the nonorganic produce appear ripe when it arrives at its destination store.

In local farmers' markets, there are some farmers who practice organic farming, but they don't have the official government certification. For smaller farms, the certification process can be too costly. If you visit a farmers' market, it is a good idea to ask the vendors about their farming practices before purchasing products. If you are lucky enough to find local farmers who practice organic farming, you have a great resource for fresh local organic produce without the high price tag. It is a winning solution for you, the farmers, and the environment.

Toxic Foods

The Environmental Working Group (EWG), headquartered in Washington, DC, is a non-profit organization dedicated to protecting human health and the environment. Its website is: https://www.ewg.org. Each year, the EWG publishes a list of the 12 most toxic fruits and vegetables (known as the "Dirty Dozen"), based on average ratings of pesticide residue on produce in North America. The EWG also publishes an annual list of the 15 cleanest nonorganic fruits and vegetables (the "Clean Fifteen"), with minimal pesticide residue. The lists for 2018 are as follows:

The Clean Fifteen – the least toxic nonorganic fruits and vegetables, from most clean to least clean

1. Avocados
2. Sweet corn
3. Pineapples

4. Cabbages
5. Onions
6. Sweet peas, frozen
7. Papayas
8. Asparagus
9. Mangoes
10. Eggplants
11. Honeydew melons
12. Kiwis
13. Cantaloupes
14. Cauliflower
15. Broccoli

The Dirty Dozen – the most toxic non-organic fruits and vegetables, from most dirty to least dirty

1. Strawberries
2. Spinach
3. Nectarines
4. Apples
5. Grapes
6. Peaches
7. Cherries
8. Pears
9. Tomatoes

10. Celery

11. Potatoes

12. Sweet bell peppers

The Clean Fifteen list is an excellent resource for people who can't always find or afford organic foods. Regarding the Dirty Dozen list, I recommend either purchasing these fruits and vegetables as organic or avoiding them entirely. For meats or other animal-based products, such as eggs and dairy, I recommend choosing organically raised meats or, at the very least, products from animals that were naturally raised. This will ensure that the animals had diets free of pesticides and other toxins that concentrate in their bodies. The more organic foods that you choose, the more reduction you will have in your personal toxicity burden. In addition, your purchases will encourage organic farmers to keep up their hard work, while sending a message to nonorganic farmers that organic is the way of the future.

Fish

How do fish fit into this discussion? Fish are an amazing source of omega-3 fatty acids and protein. Including fish frequently in your diet will help improve any conditions associated with inflammatory processes, such as endometriosis, fibromyalgia, and chronic pain. The omega-3 fatty acids from fish will also encourage the development of healthy egg quality and uterine lining, as well as improve the health of your skin.

Unfortunately, many farmed fish have the same problems as farmed animals in terms of antibiotic use and poor food quality. Another problem is that much of our fish supply is contaminated by the toxic metals and other chemical pollutants that have seeped into our waterways. The majority of large ocean fish contain high levels of toxic substances, such as mercury and polychlorinated biphenyls (PCBs). PCBs are considered persistent organic pollutants (POPs), toxic substances that resist biodegradation, remaining in the environment for long periods. ("Organic" in this sense refers to chemical compounds containing carbon.) PCBs are known to be neurotoxic (destructive to nerve tissue) and hormone-disruptive compounds, and they have been banned in the United States and Canada since 1977. Nevertheless, PCBs are still found in the environment, and they are present in high levels in many farmed fish and in fish that come from polluted bodies of water.

The following outlines the toxicity levels of commonly available fish and seafood in three categories—highly toxic, moderately toxic, and least toxic—based on average measurements of mercury and POPs. I recommend eating fish/seafood at least twice per week but sticking mainly to those in the least toxic list. For fish in the moderately toxic list, having one of these once or twice a month is acceptable. I recommend completely avoiding the fish in the highly toxic list.

Highly Toxic Fish/Seafood

Atlantic halibut, farmed salmon, grouper, king mackerel, marlin, oysters (Gulf Coast), sea bass, shark, Spanish mackerel, swordfish, tilefish (golden snapper), tuna (steaks and canned albacore)

Moderately Toxic Fish/Seafood

Alaskan halibut, American lobster, black cod, canned light tuna, freshwater bass, freshwater perch, sea trout, mahi mahi, Pacific mackerel

Least Toxic Fish/Seafood

Arctic char, anchovies, clams, crab, crayfish, farmed catfish, flounder, freshwater trout, herring, mussels, ocean perch, oysters (not Gulf Coast), Pacific flounder, Pacific sole, pike, scallops, shrimp, squid, striped bass, sturgeon, tilapia, whitefish, wild Alaska and Pacific salmon

Genetically Modified Organisms

GMOs are organisms developed through laboratory techniques that use biotechnology, such as gene splicing and other forms of genetic manipulation/engineering, to create new varieties or species of microbes, plants, and animals. The first GMO crop to be approved by the U.S. Food and Drug Administration (FDA) was a tomato with a longer shelf-life in 1994. Since then, genetically engineered varieties of corn, soya, sugar beets, canola, and other products have substantially increased in use on both Canadian and American farms.

One major concept behind the initial development of GMO crops was that genetic manipulation could make crops resistant to insects, enabling farmers to produce more product with less pesticide use, resulting in lower cost. However, this concept has been proven to be faulty. Some insects have naturally adapted to the GMO crops, meaning that farmers must use more pesticides than ever in some cases. Interestingly, many of the companies that have patents on GMO seeds are the same companies that develop and patent pesticides and herbicides.

Other concerns about GMO foods involve the unknown effects on human health of the genetically altered consumed products. There has been only limited study of the long-term safety of GMO foods on the human body. Although many scientists argue that such foods are safe, others disagree. Because of this controversy, several countries have policies requiring mandatory labeling of GMO foods. Some countries have instituted bans on both GMO food production and imports of GMO products. In 2018, the USDA unveiled guidelines for GMO labeling, which U.S. food producers will be required to follow beginning in 2020. As of 2018, Canada had not yet established labelling requirements.

The Non-GMO Project, headquartered in Bellingham, Washington, is a non-profit organization that offers voluntary certification for non-GMO food products. This organization's website is: https://www.nongmoproject.org. Farmers and food producers can use this certification labelling on their products that are not genetically modified. Since we don't know the long-term health or fertility effects of eating genetically modified foods, I believe it is best to avoid them in your diet as much as possible. Buying foods that have a government organic label or the Non-GMO Project certification will assist you in minimizing the amount of GMO foods in your diet.

Assignments

Try to raise your awareness regarding the foods that you purchase, including the source of the foods and whether the foods are organic or nonorganic and whether they are genetically modified or not genetically modified. To this end, take the following actions:

- Check if you are eating any foods on the Dirty Dozen list. If so, begin eliminating these foods from your diet and switching to organic or Clean Fifteen options. For updated lists visit https://www.ewg.org/

- Examine your fish/seafood consumption, and switch from products in the highly toxic or moderately toxic list to those in the least toxic least.

ARE EATING ORGANIC AND NON-GMO FOODS IMPORTANT?

- Seafood watch is a great website to help navigate the toxicity of various species of fish https://www.seafoodwatch.org/

- Look for foods that have certification from the Non-GMO Project.

CHAPTER 8
THE IMPORTANCE OF FATS

FATS IN THE diet are commonly considered an enemy to anyone concerned with losing weight or worried about their cardiovascular system. When an association was made between cardiovascular disease and diets high in saturated fats, people became scared to eat fatty foods. Although an excess of saturated fat is not good for us, fats in general are not bad. As the negative aspects of fats have circulated through the mass media, food manufacturers have increasingly removed fats from their products and replaced them with sugars and carbohydrates. This has led to an unfortunate consequence—the average person in North America has a diet that is deficient in essential fats and excessive in carbohydrates and sugars. The excessive carbohydrates and sugars have contributed to the skyrocketing prevalence of PCOS, type 2 diabetes mellitus, metabolic syndrome, and heart concerns.

THE IMPORTANCE OF FATS

In this chapter, you are going to learn:

- What fat is and why it is important in our diets
- The difference between good and bad fats
- Ways to add good, or healthy, fats into your diet

Fat Basics

Fat is one of the three macronutrients (dietary substances required in large amounts for life). The other categories of macronutrients are proteins and carbohydrates.

Through digestive processes, fats in your diet are broken down into fatty acids, which can then be absorbed into your bloodstream. Fatty acids build the outer membrane of every cell in your body. Your body depends on these fatty acid membranes to keep out harmful toxins and let in important nutrients. Essential fatty acids are required for maintaining proper brain function, for manufacturing hormones, and for regulating your menstrual cycle and ovulation.

We have been well trained by media reports to look for products that contain "no fat" or "low fat"—but without actually understanding which kinds of fats we want to avoid in our diet and which kinds are good for us. Not all fats are created equal and knowing the difference between fats is more important than knowing the amount of fat you eat.

Foods such as dairy products and eggs have been widely reported as causing heart disease. However, such reports contrast with the majority of major studies that have been published. Eggs are an excellent source of numerous nutrients and minerals, including protein; fat; vitamins B2, B6, B12, and D; selenium; zinc; copper; and iron. They also provide us with choline, a fat that we typically don't get enough of in our diets. Eggs are the best version of a multivitamin that you can find in nature.

Now, let's talk about the harmful fats that we want to avoid in our diets.

Trans Fats

Trans fats are found in nature in small amounts in some meat and dairy products. However, the majority of trans fats—also known as partially hydrogenated oils (PHOs)—found in our diets are synthetically made through a hydrogenation process that involves refining oils under high heat to create substances that are solid at room temperature, such as margarines. Trans fats are commonly found in many food products, including breakfast cereals, crackers, chips, microwave popcorn, cakes, cookies, doughnuts, biscuits, frozen pizza, and fried fast foods. Trans fats give food products longer shelf lives, so they are usually present in packaged and processed foods.

Trans fats have been directly linked to damage in the cardiovascular system. These substances act to increase levels of your "bad" cholesterol (low-density lipoprotein [LDL] cholesterol) and lower levels of your "good" cholesterol (high-density lipoprotein [HDL] cholesterol). They also impair your immune function and have a negative impact on your fertility. It has been estimated that trans fats have approximately five times more negative impact on the body than saturated fats.

Because of the well-documented harmful effects of trans fats on human health, there have been many efforts to remove these substances from food products. In the United States, the FDA announced in 2015 that it does not recognize manufactured trans fats as safe, and the agency gave manufacturers three years to remove them from all food products. As of June 2018, manufacturers had to ensure that products sold in the United States did not contain PHOs for any uses that have not been approved by the FDA. In Canada, there is a voluntary system in which companies are left to decide whether they want to remove trans fats from their products. However, manufacturers are required to list the amounts of trans fats on food labelling, so be sure to read the fats section of nutrition labels. Certain terms, such as partially hydrogenated oils and vegetable oil shortening, indicate that the product contains trans fats. If you see trans fats listed, you would be wise to avoid the product.

Saturated Fats

Saturated fats can be a little confusing to consider. There are two types of saturated fats—long-chain and short-chain. Long-chain saturated fats are solid at room temperature and include some fats in animal products, such as meat and dairy products. Too many of these saturated fats in the diet can promote inflammation and increase the risk of heart disease.

Short-chain saturated fats are found in butter, coconut oil, and various other products. These fats do not clog your arteries or contribute to heart disease. Short-chain saturated fats are easy for your body to digest and use as a fuel source.

Saturated fats from either plant or animal sources provide the building blocks for cell membranes and for a variety of hormones. For this reason, they should never be eliminated from your diet. If your diet is deficient in saturated fats, you will not be able to adequately generate cholesterol, which is necessary to make all your hormones.

Unsaturated Fats

Unsaturated fats are classified as omega-3, omega-6, and omega-9 fats. As we previously noted in the chapter on supplements, both omega-3 and omega-6 fats are considered to be essential fatty acids—meaning that they need to be consumed in the diet because your body can't make them. Active forms of both omega-3 and omega-6 fats are responsible for regulating several processes in the body, including inflammation, blood clotting, and blood vessel dilation.

You want to aim for a diet that has no trans fats, with approximately 30 percent of your fat coming from sources of saturated fat, mainly meats. The remainder of your fat consumption should come from unsaturated fats, with a focus on omega-3 fatty acids.

Healthy Fat Sources

What foods should you consume to get more of the healthy fatty acids in your diet? Use the following list as a guide:

- Avocado
- Beef (lean)
- Chicken
- Eggs (whole)
- Fish (fatty), such as salmon, herring, anchovies, sardines
- Nuts, such as almonds, cashews, macadamia, walnuts
- Oils, such as extra virgin olive, coconut, flax, or grapeseed
- Seeds, such as flax, chia, pumpkin, sesame,
- Turkey

Try to get four to six servings of these nutritious fat-rich foods in your daily diet. Examples of a serving size include: half an avocado, one-quarter cup of nuts or seeds, one teaspoon of oils, two eggs, and three ounces of fatty fish or animal meats (about the size of your palm). You should be sure to have a fat source at each meal. This could be as simple as using olive oil or coconut oil for cooking. Many of the healthy fat-rich foods are also high in protein, so you can cover both dietary requirements with one food. It never ceases to amaze me how clever Mother Nature is! If you would like more support my enhance fertility bootcamp program you will receive recipes and online support.

Assignments

- Adjust your diet to get four to six servings of the previously described healthy fat-rich foods daily, with at least three of the servings from non-animal sources.

- Check your cupboards for processed foods that contain either trans fats or high amounts of saturated fats. Discard these foods or make a mental note to no longer purchase them.

- Record the items in your diet for a few days. Then review the items to check if you are getting the necessary fats daily. If not, make dietary adjustments.

- For further recipes and dietary support please join our community at https://enhancefertility.ca/ and on Facebook or Instagram @Enhancefertility

CHAPTER 9
CARBOHYDRATES ARE NOT THE ENEMY

CARBOHYDRATES ARE THE second macronutrient, after fats, that we are focusing on. The next will be proteins. In recent years, we have seen various popular diets that eliminate or drastically reduce the amount of consumed carbohydrates. Such diets can be harmful to your health and adversely affect your fertility.

In this chapter, we will cut through the popular misinformation to shed light on the following issues:

- The impact of carbohydrates on insulin levels
- The role of carbohydrates in the inflammatory process
- The food sources of carbohydrates, and the role of these sources in fertility

Carbohydrates and Insulin

Carbohydrates are an essential part of our diet. They are necessary for energy production and brain function. The optimal function of all your organs and muscles depends on stable levels of sugars, which are carbohydrates, in your bloodstream.

Carbohydrates include all forms of sugars, from both complex and simple sources. Complex carbohydrates are obtained from foods such as brown rice, whole wheat, rye, sweet potatoes, squash, and beans. Simple sugars are obtained from fruits and any sources of refined grains, such as white bread, pasta, white rice, cookies, and pastries.

When you consume a food containing complex carbohydrates, the compounds are broken down in the digestive process into simple sugars, such as glucose and sucrose. These sugars are absorbed into your bloodstream, triggering your pancreas to release a hormone called insulin. The insulin attaches to receptors on your cells, allowing the sugars to move from the bloodstream into the cells. Your body will adjust the amount of insulin it secretes based on the amount of carbohydrates and sugars you consume.

Insulin controls blood sugar levels, but it also promotes the inflammatory process. Problems with the body's insulin production or insulin use are associated with increased inflammation and infertility, as well as a host of chronic diseases, including heart disease, diabetes, and cancer. The less insulin we need to secrete, the better. As we age, or if we consistently eat large amounts of carbohydrates, our cell receptors can become less sensitive to insulin. This means that the body has to produce even more insulin to keep blood sugar levels stable. This condition is known as insulin resistance and is common in women who have higher percentages of body fat and in women with PCOS. Insulin resistance is usually the first stage of progression to type-2 diabetes.

In the typical North American diet, carbohydrates constitute upwards of 60 percent of the calories consumed. The amount of refined sugar (processed simple sugar) in the diet has gone through the roof during the past few decades. Simple, refined sugars are problematic in our diet because they cause the fastest and sharpest spikes in insulin levels. Such sugars are found in the majority of packaged foods, so eating a diet high in processed foods leads to a greater amount of sugar in the bloodstream. Sugar tastes great and is highly addictive, which is why it is so difficult to remove from our diets.

Carbohydrates and Fertility

There have been studies showing that the success rate of in vitro fertilization (IVF) increases when women have a diet relatively low in carbohydrates and relatively high in proteins. It has also been demonstrated that embryos have a challenging time thriving in an environment that is high in sugar.

In a study by Jeffrey B. Russell, MD, of the Delaware Institute of Reproductive Medicine, researchers evaluated the impacts of diets containing high or low levels of carbohydrates and proteins in different groups of women undergoing IVF[17]. For the group of women who had a diet of at least 25-percent protein, 64 percent of the women experienced development of a blastocyst (early embryo), compared with 34 percent of the women in the low-protein group. The clinical pregnancy rate was 67 percent in the high-protein group versus 32 percent in the low-protein group. Pregnancy rates improved further when the diet was made up of less than 40-percent carbohydrates and at least 25-percent protein. Those women achieved clinical pregnancy rates of 80 percent.

Reducing Simple Sugars in the Diet

You should get more of your carbohydrates from complex sources, and fewer from simple sources. Thus, you need to identify where sugars are in your diet. If you are eating any packaged foods, sugar will appear in the ingredient list under a variety of names, including sucrose, glucose, fructose, maltose, lactose, dextrose, high fructose corn syrup, corn syrup solids, cane juice, dextrin, fruit juice concentrate, raw sugar, rice syrup, syrup, and treacle. All of these variations of sugar will produce the same impact on your body—increasing blood sugar levels and causing a dump of insulin into the bloodstream.

High fructose corn syrup is one of the worst sugars. It is the type of sweetener found in soda and many processed foods. It can adversely affect the liver's ability to detoxify the blood, and it can contribute to fatty liver disease. I recommend completely eliminating high fructose corn syrup from your diet. Ideally, it would be best to remove all sugars mentioned in the previous paragraph. At the very least, you should make sure that they are not your primary source of carbohydrate fuel.

There are several alternative and healthier sweetener options that you can use in place of sugar. These include stevia, dates, apple butter, coconut sugar, berries, and honey. I do not recommend using artificial sweeteners, like aspartame or sucralose, because these have their own set of health concerns. It is best to stick to the naturally occurring options.

Grains and Gluten

Other than refined sugars, the other sources of carbohydrates that can be highly problematic are grains. Wheat is a gluten-containing grain that is found in most of our baked goods, such as breads, bagels, doughnuts, pastries, muffins, and pasta. There has been a steady increase over the past two decades in the development of wheat sensitivities and an autoimmune condition called celiac disease, in which wheat and all gluten-containing grains cause damage to the intestinal tract. Undiagnosed celiac disease can be the cause of infertility in both men and women.

Wheat is one of the most highly processed grains on the market. In our modern-day society, wheat has been greatly modified compared to the wheat that our ancestors ate. Today's processed wheat contains a significantly higher amount of gluten, which makes it harder to digest. This is likely the reason that wheat causes so many health concerns today.

Gluten is a protein that is found in high amounts in wheat. It is also found in other grains, including rye, spelt, and barley. Some people find that they feel significantly better without any gluten in their diet. Other people find that wheat is the main problematic grain, and the other gluten-containing grains do not bother them. Symptoms associated with a wheat or gluten sensitivity include anemia, abdominal pain, headaches, ear infections, eczema, bloating and gas, depression and anxiety, diarrhea and constipation, fatigue and weakness, impaired thyroid function, infertility or multiple miscarriages, aching joints or overall body soreness, and inflammation. Any of these symptoms may indicate gluten intolerance.

Research findings and clinical experience have revealed many interesting aspects of the effects of gluten and wheat on health. These findings are summarized in the following points.

- Consumption of modern wheat by people with weakened immune systems may trigger or contribute to autoimmune diseases, such as type-1 diabetes mellitus, rheumatoid arthritis, Crohn's disease, Hashimoto's disease, and multiple sclerosis.
- Wheat can increase acidic conditions in the body, countering the more alkaline pH balance that is beneficial

for health and fertility. Thus, wheat might throw you off your goal of getting pregnant.

- Gluten sensitivity contributes to chronic inflammation throughout the body. Inflammation is a cause of concern for women with PCOS, endometriosis, and any autoimmune condition. In such cases, eating gluten will often exacerbate the problem.

- Infertility seems to be more common in women with untreated celiac disease or gluten sensitivity. These women may also be more at risk for recurrent miscarriages and preterm births.

- A gluten-free diet may help women with endometriosis symptoms. For many of my patients, excluding wheat for two or three cycles has resulted in reductions in pain levels. It is worthwhile to see if this approach makes a difference in your pain during periods and ovulation.

- Wheat and most other grains sold in North America are fortified with synthetic folic acid. About 20 percent of the population is unable to properly metabolize folic acid, leading to impairment of an important chemical process called methylation. Problems with this process can affect the reproductive system and other systems of the body, as is discussed in chapter 17 Genes and Fertility.

- Another bonus to giving up wheat is that it is one of the quickest ways to lose weight, often to astounding degrees! I have also observed that patients who drop wheat from their diets experience relief of acid reflux and bowel urgency, elimination of joint pain, reversal of eczema and other skin rashes, and reduction of depression and anxiety.

Sugar from Fruits

Fruits contain a type of simple sugar called fructose. Different fruits have varying amounts of sugar content. Fruits with lower fructose levels include berries, cherries, apples, and pears. Fruits with higher fructose levels include grapes, pineapples, bananas, and papaya. I generally recommend eating those fruits that have lower amounts of fructose—fruits lower on the glycemic index. It is advisable to limit consumption of the higher-fructose fruits. Even with naturally occurring sugars, you can get too much of a good thing. Ideally, you should have between two and four servings of fruits daily.

Best Carbohydrates to Consume

When you hear all the confusing and contradictory misinformation about carbohydrates in the media, keep the following points in mind. They will serve as guidelines for getting the best carbohydrates in your diet.

- It is ideal to get your carbohydrates mostly from unrefined natural sources, especially such vegetables as sweet potatoes, squashes, beets, and cauliflower.
- Beans and legumes, such as lentils or chickpeas, are good sources of both proteins and carbohydrates.
- Fruits that are lower in sugars, such as berries, cherries, apples, pears, and pomegranates, are the best fruit sources of carbohydrates.
- Certain seeds, such as sesame, pumpkin, and chia, are good sources of carbohydrates as well as protein and healthy fats.

- Healthy grains that don't contain gluten include brown or wild rice, gluten-free oats, quinoa, buckwheat, and amaranth.

- If you love to bake, use flours made from any of the grains listed above, or use nut flours, such as almond flour.

Assignments

- Try eliminating refined sugars and gluten-containing grains from your diet for the next three weeks. During this time, see if you notice any changes with your health or mood, such as changes in your digestive system, skin, sleep patterns, or energy levels.

- Focus on getting most of your carbohydrates from starchy vegetables (such as sweet potatoes and beets), beans and lentils, low-fructose fruits, and non-gluten grains.

- As you adjust your diet, keep the following points in mind. When you first eliminate sugars or other foods that you are used to, you will generally have cravings for these foods for about three or four days. The cravings can be intense. During this time, the cravings can be curbed by eating higher amounts of low fructose fruits or dried fruits. If you stay strong, the cravings will subside, and you will start to feel considerably better. It will be easier to stick to your healthier diet if you don't have any of the problematic foods readily available in your home!

CHAPTER 10
THE IMPORTANCE OF PROTEIN

IN THIS CHAPTER, we are going to discuss our third macronutrient, protein, and examine its importance for conception. Of all the macronutrients, which also include fats and carbohydrates, protein is the only one that the body does not store. Therefore, it must be consumed in the diet on a regular basis.

Protein is the basic building block for all living cells, and it is required to maintain, heal, and repair our tissues. It is also a building block of hormones, enzymes, and blood. Eating protein at each meal helps to stabilize blood sugar levels, which helps to reduce food cravings. Proteins usually take between three and five hours to digest, which is how they keep you feeling full longer and how they minimize sugar cravings. Adequate protein consumption and the resulting blood sugar balance are crucial when it comes to healthy fertility.

At the end of this chapter, you will understand the following:

- The food sources of proteins
- The amount of protein you should be eating daily, and how to calculate this amount
- The role of protein in conception

Sources of Protein

The best sources of protein are fish, lean meats, beans, lentils, peas, soy, quinoa, nuts, seeds and eggs.

Dairy products from cows are also a source of protein. However, many people have difficulty digesting such products, which can promote inflammation in these individuals. Because of this possibility, it may be better to avoid dairy products as a protein source. If you are going to consume dairy products, full-fat products are preferable to no-fat or low-fat options in terms of optimal fertility.

Knowing which proteins to eat and when to eat them can get confusing. Meat and other animal sources of protein can be more acidic for the body than plant sources. But proteins from animal sources are "complete," while plant proteins are not. In other words, animal proteins contain all the essential amino acids, which the body needs to function. Considering all these issues, it is a good idea to consume a combination of plant and animal sources of protein. If your preference is to eat a vegan or vegetarian based diet, you need to be more vigilant about ensuring you get enough protein and all your essential amino acids in your daily diet.

In order to curb cravings and keep blood sugar balanced in the bloodstream, it is ideal to include protein in each meal or snack. Remember that protein is the main macronutrient that makes you feel full and satisfied.

Amounts of Protein

The amount of protein that you should consume depends on your weight. To calculate this amount of protein, you can multiply your weight in pounds by 0.36, or your weight in kilograms by 0.8. This calculation gives you your daily protein requirement in grams (g). For the average female, this is approximately 46 g of protein per day. This essentially works out to about 15 g of protein per meal if you are eating the recommended three meals per day. For some women, a diet higher in protein may be advisable, to help them maintain a healthy weight and body fat percentage. For these women, daily protein intake in the range of 80 to 100 g helps to improve satiety and control of blood sugar levels. Women who have a difficult time with sugar cravings or who have concerns with blood sugar regulation such as PCOS or type 2 diabetes would fall into this category.

To aid in your dietary planning, the following list provides the amounts of protein in grams, as found in some common sources:

- 3 oz chicken breast = 27 g
- 3 oz turkey = 22 g
- 3 oz salmon = 21 g
- 3 oz roast beef = 19 g
- 1 cup lentils = 18 g
- 1 cup legumes/beans = 14.5 g
- 1 cup cooked quinoa = 9 g

THE IMPORTANCE OF PROTEIN

- ¼ cup raw almonds = 8 g
- 1 cup broccoli = 6 g
- 1 cup soy milk = 9 g
- 1 large egg = 6 g

Assignments

- Using the equation described in this chapter, calculate the amount of daily protein you should be consuming based on your body weight.
- Monitor the protein sources in your diet for a few days. Calculate the amount of protein that you are getting at each meal and add up the amounts from all meals and snacks during the day. If you aren't getting a protein source at each meal and if you aren't getting a minimum of about 50 g daily (or your weight-based calculated amount), adjust your diet accordingly.
- As you increase your protein intake, note if you are observing improved consistency in your energy, mood, and hormonal regulation.

CHAPTER 11
THE BENEFITS OF SMOOTHIES

SMOOTHIES CAN BE a great way to increase the number of fruits and vegetables in your diet. They also serve as a good source of fats and protein.

In this chapter, you will learn:

- Why smoothies are healthy for you
- Ingredients that should go into your smoothies, and ingredients that you should skip

What are Smoothies?

Smoothies can serve as either a meal or a snack, depending on what ingredients you put into them.

I have found that even patients who generally adhere to healthy diets can have difficulty reaching the optimal amount of seven to ten servings of fruits and vegetables daily. On

THE BENEFITS OF SMOOTHIES

average, only 14 percent of North Americans achieve the five-serving daily minimum. Blending is a wonderful way to pack more leafy greens into your diet, especially for people who may not find these vegetables very tasty. Adding greens also adds fiber, which is essential for keeping your system clean and running smoothly.

Smoothies allow you to add a variety of produce to your diet. This alkalinizes the body, aids in tissue healing, reduces inflammation (the root cause of most chronic diseases), delivers nutrients to your cells, enhances brain function, improves hormonal balance, balances blood sugars, and improves digestion.

Smoothies can help your body by increasing your consumption of vitamins and minerals, fiber, and antioxidants.

- The vitamins and minerals in smoothies come from food sources that are easy for the body to absorb. These vitamins and minerals include zinc, calcium, selenium, iron, folic acid, and vitamins A, C, and E. These and other nutrients in smoothies are necessary for regulating your monthly cycle, ovulation, and healthy fertility.

- Fiber is an important part of a healthy diet and essential for healthy hormonal balance. The important roles of fiber include ridding the body of excess hormones, balancing blood sugar levels, and enhancing digestion.

- Antioxidants are involved in chemical reactions that prevent cell damage in the body, and they play a role in the quality of both eggs and sperm. For a couple trying to conceive, smoothies can be a great way to increase your antioxidant intake.

Making a Smoothie

If you are new to the world of smoothies, the first thing you will need is a blender. For optimal blending, use a high-powered blender, which will do a better job breaking up the greens and other vegetables. Then you will need certain food products to put into the blender. Combine all the ingredients and blend until smooth. If your smoothie is meant to replace a meal, it should contain the following basic ingredients:

- Water, coconut water, or nut or soy milk
- 1 to 2 cups of greens
- ½ to 1 cup of fruits or sweet vegetables
- 1 to 2 tablespoons of a plant-based fat source, such as coconut oil, avocado, or flax seeds
- 1 to 2 tablespoons of a plant-based protein source, such as protein powder (from soy, hemp, brown rice, peas, or pumpkin seeds), chia seeds, sesame seeds, or seed or nut butters
- Your supplements can also be added to smoothies to decrease the number of capsules you need to swallow.

The amazing thing about smoothies is that there are countless variations of ingredients, and you can change them as often as you like. Having a smoothie for breakfast is a great way to avoid the grains and sugars that can be problematic carbohydrates. Below are a few sample smoothie recipes to get you started.

Green Smoothie
1 banana (peeled)
1 scoop protein powder
2 organic kale leaves

1.5 cups filtered water
2 tbsp organic almond butter
1 pinch cinnamon
1 tbsp coconut oil
4 ice cubes

Antioxidant Smoothie
1 cup almond milk
3 cups organic fresh spinach
1 tbsp coconut oil
1/2 cup cherries, pitted (fresh or frozen)
1/2 cup blueberries (fresh or frozen)
1 tbsp raw cacao powder

Chocolate Lover's Smoothie
2 kale leaves
1/2 frozen banana
1 tbsp almond butter
1 scoop protein powder
1 tbsp cacao nibs
1-2 cups filtered water

Tropical Smoothie
2 kale leaves
1/2 banana
1/2 cup strawberries
1/2 cup pineapple, cubed (fresh or frozen)
1 scoop protein powder
2 cups water
1 tbsp hemp and/or flaxseeds

Assignments

- If you haven't had a smoothie before, try making one this weekend.
- For more smoothie and recipe support consider sign up for the mailing list at Enhance Fertility to receive your free recipe book https://enhancefertility.ca/ and speak with your nutritionist or naturopathic doctor

CHAPTER 12
HOW TO IMPROVE EGG/ OOCYTE QUALITY

THE FOCUS OF this chapter is the importance of the quality of your oocytes (immature eggs) and your ova (mature eggs) in your ability to conceive, as well as in optimizing the health of your future baby.

As a woman, you were born with all the oocytes that you will ever have—all the potential eggs that you will ever produce. As you age, all the cells in your body start to show damage, and your eggs are no exception. Older women tend to produce less viable eggs. The environment in which your oocytes mature into ova can be modified through diet and lifestyle factors. Optimizing the nutrients that are in your follicular fluid, surrounding your developing eggs, will have a positive impact on the health of your eggs. It takes about three months for a developing egg to progress from its primordial cell state to the point of ovulation. Thus, you should use this time to make your internal environment as healthy as possible to encourage and enhance healthy egg development.

This chapter will cover the following topics as guidance for optimizing your egg quality:

- Health of mitochondria
- Immune function
- Free-radical status of follicular fluid
- Nutrients and supplements that positively impact egg quality

Body Systems

There are three body systems that are worth focusing on regarding the health and quality of a woman's oocytes and ova. These systems involve the mitochondria, immune function, and free radicals in follicular fluid.

1. Mitochondria are organelles that are found in every cell of the body. Egg cells contain a high concentration of mitochondria. These organelles produce energy for your cells, allowing the cells to function efficiently. As we age and as we are increasingly exposed to toxins, our mitochondria become less efficient and they produce less energy. Insufficient energy production can have a negative impact on the body's ability to detoxify itself and protect its DNA (deoxyribonucleic acid, the molecule that makes up genes).

    Mitochondria are very susceptible to toxins, which is one reason that toxic substances may play a huge role in a woman's fertility status. It is possible that toxicity, which is not routinely evaluated, is responsible some cases of unexplained infertility. We will cover this topic in more detail in Chapter 16 – The Role of Hormone-Disrupting Toxins in Fertility.

2. Cells of the immune system secrete an enzyme called myeloperoxidase (MPO). This enzyme is found in higher levels when there is severe inflammation, and it has been directly linked to poor egg quality and poor reproductive outcomes. This is one of the reasons that chronic inflammation and autoimmune conditions, such as Hashimoto's thyroiditis, can play big roles in infertility.

   The immune system has two main, general types of cells—T cells and B cells. Studies have shown that many patients with endometriosis have low numbers of a type of T cell called T regulatory cells. Somewhere between 25 percent and 50 percent of women with infertility have endometriosis. The exact percentage is uncertain because endometriosis often goes undiagnosed. Whatever the percentage, immune imbalance is clearly relevant to a considerable number of couples.

3. Free radicals can arise in the body through normal detoxification and metabolic processes. They can also enter the body as toxins from the air or the water and food you consume. If your body doesn't have enough resources to neutralize the free radicals, they can cause damage to any of the cells in the body. When free radicals are found at elevated levels in the follicular fluid, which surrounds your developing eggs, they can damage or negatively impact your egg quality.

Nutrients and Supplements

There are several nutrients that are beneficial to egg quality. Many dietary considerations that can affect egg cells and fertility have previously been discussed in this book. However, if you are over age 35 or have had failed IVF cycles because of poor egg quality, you may benefit from certain supplements.

Laboratory research and clinical findings indicate that certain nutrients play roles in improving the quality of your eggs through mechanisms involving mitochondrial function, immune function, and/or free-radical status. These nutrients, available as supplements, are described in the following text, along with research findings about them. If you are interested in reading more details on this research, please refer to the cited references. You do not need to add all of these substances to your routine. However, I want to bring them to your attention so that you are aware of the variety of nutrients available for improving egg quality, depending on your individual situation.

Myo-inositol

Myo-inositol is in the B vitamin family. It forms part of your cell membrane and is involved in sugar and hormonal regulation. It is also important in fertility, because it enhances the development of mature eggs and improves the chances of egg fertilization. Myo-inositol concentrates in the follicular fluid, and there is a direct relationship between its concentration and egg quality. Its role has been examined in multiple studies of women with fertility concerns. One study correlated intake of myo-inositol with improvement in the following areas:

- Increased clinical pregnancy rates
- Improved number of high-quality eggs
- Higher number of retrieved eggs

- Decrease in number of immature eggs

The ideal dose of myo-inositol found in the studies was between 1 and 4 g/day[18] . In addition, clinical trials using myo-inositol in women with PCOS showed regular ovulation in women who had not previously ovulated. In most studies of women with PCOS, a dose of 4 g/day was found to be optimal[19].

Melatonin

Melatonin, a hormone secreted by the pineal gland in the brain, is best known for its impact on promoting sleep. Melatonin also acts as an antioxidant, reducing the oxidative stress on tissue caused by free radicals. It naturally increases during ovulation to help protect the eggs.

In addition, melatonin plays an important role in egg maturation. Studies have found that supplements of low-dose melatonin (1-3 mg) enhanced egg maturation. Both laboratory and clinical studies have demonstrated that melatonin can improve the health of eggs and embryos.

Studies investigating the combination of melatonin and myo-inositol have documented improvements in egg and embryo quality, as well as in other variables. The combination was shown to reduce the adverse effects (side effects) associated with such medicated procedures as IVF. This is especially important for women with PCOS, whose cycles tend to get hyper-stimulated in IVF[20].

Alpha-Lipoic Acid

Alpha-lipoic acid (ALA) is a powerful antioxidant. Its effects, in combination with those of myo-inositol, have been studied in women with PCOS who were undergoing IVF. The data suggested that the combination helped to improve reproductive outcomes, as well as metabolism in general. Researchers found that after three months, the combination of ALA and myo-inositol led to an improvement in egg quality. The data provided support for the use of this long-term combination in the prevention of PCOS[21].

Coenzyme Q10

Coenzyme Q10 (CoQ10) is a naturally occurring antioxidant made by your body. This antioxidant is important for mitochondrial health, which, in turn, is important for fertility. As you age, there is a decline in function of the enzymes that make CoQ10. This can be associated with fertility problems. In studies of lab animals with poor mitochondrial function, administration of CoQ10 prevented premature ovarian failure. These results suggested that impaired mitochondrial performance caused by low CoQ10 availability may contribute to age-associated egg deficits and infertility.

Another study investigated the combination of 60 mg of CoQ10 daily, in combination with a common fertility medication called clomiphene citrate[22]. The investigators concluded that the combination improved ovulation cycles and clinical pregnancies, compared with the use of clomiphene alone. The typical dose of CoQ10, that has been found to aid fertility, is 200 to 600 mg/day.

N-acetylcysteine and L-carnitine

N-acetylcysteine (NAC) is an amino-acid building block for an antioxidant made in the liver called glutathione. Nutritional support for glutathione production will help reduce the amount of damage caused by free radicals.

One study examined the use of NAC, metformin, or a combination of both for women with PCOS who were undergoing intracytoplasmic sperm injections (ICSI). The women in the study received NAC (600 mg three times per day), metformin (1500 mg/day), a combination of both, or a placebo for six weeks. Their oocytes were then retrieved for analysis. Results showed that the number of immature and abnormal oocytes decreased significantly in the NAC group, while the number of good-quality embryos was higher in the NAC group, compared to the placebo group. The researchers concluded that NAC improves the quality of oocytes and embryos, making it a viable alternative to metformin[23].

Another study looked at the use of NAC in combination with an amino acid called L-carnitine to prevent DNA damage in the eggs of infertile women with mild endometriosis. The researchers found that the use of NAC and L-carnitine together can prevent the egg damage that is caused by free radicals[24]. L-carnitine benefits mitochondrial function by transporting fuel, in the form of fatty acids, from the bloodstream to the mitochondria. If mitochondria don't receive enough fatty acids, they are unable to produce sufficient energy for cells to function optimally. L-carnitine is also an important consideration if you are supplementing with CoQ10, because CoQ10 can't get into the mitochondria to do its work if you are deficient in L-carnitine. L-carnitine is found in animal protein sources. If you are a vegetarian or taking CoQ10 in doses higher then 200 mg, it is best to add supplemental L-carnitine to ensure that you derive the maximum beneficial effects from CoQ10. L-carnitine should be dosed between 1,000 and 2,000 mg/day.

Vitamins C and E

Vitamins C and E are both antioxidants that can help to clear potentially damaging free radicals from the follicular fluid. Vitamin E also assists in thickening the uterine lining by encouraging more blood flow. These two vitamins can be found in good-quality prenatal supplements, as well as in diets rich in fruits and vegetables. Vitamin E occurs in highest amounts in foods such as avocados, tomatoes, wheat germ, and unrefined vegetable oils. If your diet is not providing enough vitamin E, try using the mixed tocopherol supplement form, up to 400IU/day. Vitamin C supplements should usually be dosed at 1-2 g/day.

Additional Notes

I have had a number of patients over the years who were struggling with recurrent miscarriages or failed IVF attempts. After supplementing with various combinations of the nutrients discussed in this chapter, they went on to have healthy pregnancies and healthy babies. I realize that this chapter presents a wealth of information about several studies and their findings on supplements. If you are left feeling overwhelmed and still have questions about supplements, joining the Facebook group Enhance fertility or consulting with your health professional is a great idea.

If you haven't yet been diagnosed with a specific fertility condition, the most important area to focus on would be your mitochondrial health. This would mainly involve supplementing with CoQ10, L-carnitine, NAC, and ALA. Remember that a baby receives all its mitochondria from the mother's egg—and none from the sperm. The health of the mother's mitochondria is extremely important. Deficits in mitochondrial function have been linked to a host of health concerns, including fibromyalgia, chronic fatigue, autism spectrum disorder, depression, anxiety, cancer, and heart disease. The healthier you can make your mitochondria as a potential mother, the better it will be for both your health and that of your future children.

Assignments

- If you are under age 35 and preparing for a healthy pregnancy, you may not need to add any supplemental support for egg quality. But if you are over age 35, or if you have been having difficulty conceiving, review the information in this chapter and consider adding the discussed supplements to support healthy egg development. Discuss this issue with your healthcare provider.

- Take at look at https://enhancefertility.ca/ for more articles on egg health

CHAPTER 13
OPTIMIZING SPERM HEALTH

MEN, NOW IT'S your turn. In this chapter, we are going to discuss how to optimize the health of sperm. Sperm makes up half of the equation for your baby, so it is extremely important for this part of conception not to be overlooked.

In this chapter we will focus on the following topics:

- Testing of sperm
- Optimizing lifestyle to encourage healthy sperm production
- Supplements for improving the health of sperm

Sperm Analysis

Infertility has traditionally been thought of as a concern that affects only women. However, it is now well-established that about one-third of infertility cases are actually due to the male factor.

If you have been trying to conceive for over a year without success, both partners should get a clinical workup done with a fertility expert. For the male partner, this workup includes a sperm analysis. There are several parameters that can be evaluated during a sperm analysis. They are all important to giving a realistic and accurate picture about the health of your sperm.

Before providing your sperm sample, it is important that you remain abstinent for two or three days (this includes both intercourse and masturbation). If you have ejaculated less than two days before your analysis, your sperm count can appear artificially low. If the last ejaculation occurred more than four days before the analysis, the quality of the test may be questionable. Because sperm only live for a few days, the sample will contain a lot of non-viable sperm.

It is also important that the sperm sample be fresh. Ideally, the sample should be produced at the site where it will be tested. For men who have difficulty with this, please speak to your lab. Most labs will be able to provide a container for you to collect the sample at home, but you must deliver it to the lab within about an hour of collection.

The sample will typically be tested for the following parameters:

1. Count (total number of sperm)
2. Motility (how well the sperm can swim)
3. Morphology (how they look, normally each with one head and one tail)
4. pH (degree of acidity or alkalinity)
5. Total volume of fluid

6. Agglutination (how sticky they are)

7. MAR test (for antibodies)

Let's examine each of these parameters, and then discuss what can be done about any concerns that may arise.

1. **Count.** Sperm count, measured in million per millilitre (mL), is usually described as having a healthy range with a lower end of 15 million/mL. The average count is about 60 million/mL. However, I generally go with the "more is better" approach. For men with counts under 30 million/mL, there is a strong possibility that this relatively low count is a contributor to infertility concerns.

   Common causes of low sperm count include the following:

   - Infections
   - Stress
   - Hormonal imbalances
   - Heat exposure
   - Excessive exercise
   - Steroid use
   - Age
   - Drug use
   - Environmental toxins
   - Genetic factors

   Research has demonstrated that changes made to diet and lifestyle can play significant roles in improving sperm counts.

2. **Motility.** The motility results, given as percentages, indicate how well the sperm can move. One result provides the total percentage of sperm that are moving. The other result provides the percentage of sperm that are swimming forward. These figures should, at minimum, be 40% for total movement and 32% for forward motion. If the sperm can't move forward, there is very little chance that they will be able to meet the egg for fertilization.

   Causes of poor motility, which are similar to those of poor count, involve the following:

   - Age
   - Weight
   - Drug use
   - Infections
   - Heat exposure
   - Excessive exercise
   - Steroid use
   - Zinc deficiency
   - Anti-sperm antibodies
   - Defects in the sperm's tails
   - Longer length of time between ejaculations

   As with sperm count, there is much research suggesting that lifestyle and dietary changes can improve sperm motility.

3. **Morphology.** The morphology parameter refers to how the sperm actually look, with the result reported based

on the percentage of sperm that appear to be normal. Different labs use different parameters to assess morphology, but up to 96% of sperm can appear abnormal and a sperm sample can still be deemed as healthy. Having a poor count or motility in combination with a high percentage of abnormal sperm, means that few sperm are going to have the ability to make their way to the egg. If the percentage of abnormal sperm is greater than 96%, your specialist will likely recommend a process called intracytoplasmic sperm injection (ICSI). In this process, sperms cells are injected directly into egg cells obtained through IVF.

The causes of poor morphology are similar to those for poor counts. However, my clinical experience suggests that environmental toxins play an especially significant role in poor morphology. I often see male patients with morphology problems who work in environments with significant toxic exposure, such as mechanics, firefighters, and chemical plant operators.

Research indicates that certain supplements, including CoQ10, can be effective in improving morphology, as well as count and motility.

4. **pH.** The pH of healthy semen is slightly alkaline, between 7.2 and 8.0 on the pH scale. The pH of semen is determined by the fluids that come from the seminal vesicles and the prostate. A pH result that is too high or too low may indicate a problem with one of these glands.

5. **Total volume.** After two or three days of not ejaculating, the total volume of semen should be about 1.5 mL or more. As with the pH, since most of the fluid comes from glands around the testicles, a low volume can point to concerns with one of these areas.

6. **Agglutination.** The agglutination test essentially reveals how sticky the sperm is and how much of the sperm is sticking together. If there are several sperm cells clumped together, this makes it less likely like the sperm will be able to swim to meet the egg. Generally, there is increased agglutination in men who have higher levels of antibodies in their sperm (discussed further in the following MAR section).

7. **MAR test.** The MAR (mixed agglutination reaction) test indicates the number of antibodies that are attacking the sperm. If more than 50% of the sperm cells are coated in antibodies, a procedure called intrauterine insemination (IUI) will typically be suggested. In IUI, sperm is inserted directly into the uterus with a catheter. If more than 80% of the sperm have antibodies, ICSI is usually recommended. There are also dietary and lifestyle changes that can help reduce antibodies and improve this parameter.

Lifestyle Changes

There are a number of basic lifestyle changes that can help to improve the overall health of the sperm. Some of these changes may seem obvious. Nevertheless, if you are not currently following these suggestions, I urge you to start now. These are healthy lifestyle practices regardless of whether your sperm parameters are good or poor.

- Stop smoking. Evidence shows that smoking damages the DNA in sperm. Damaged DNA means the sperm will be less successful at creating a healthy embryo.

- Be careful about overheating the testicles. This means that you should limit hot tub use, wear loose-fitting clothing, and avoid prolonged sitting.

- Make sure that you ejaculate regularly, at least twice per week.

- Reduce your stress levels. Performing mindfulness/meditation for 10 minutes daily can help reduce levels of stress hormones.

- Exercise regularly but not excessively. If pregnancy is the goal, this is not the time to start Ironman training. Excessive exercise can divert testosterone away from the testicles.

- Don't carry your cell phone in your pants' pocket or sit with a computer on your lap. It is possible that these practices could lead to DNA damage in the sperm.

- Get screened for sexually transmitted diseases to make sure you don't have any infections that may impact sperm health.

- Moderate your alcohol intake, to four or fewer drinks per week

- Check your caffeine intake and keep to a maximum of two cups of coffee per day.

- Reduce your toxin burden (to be discussed in Chapter 16).

- Clean up your diet. Implement the recommendations from the nutrition focussed chapters. The more you focus on fruits and vegetables, lean proteins, and healthy fats, the better your overall health and the better your sperm health. Keep in mind that the chapters on nutrition apply to both partners.

It takes about three months for your sperm to develop, similar to a woman's eggs. However, the difference between the genders is that the sperm cells are newly developed, unlike the primordial egg cells that women are born with. Because a man is constantly making new sperm, diet and lifestyle can play key roles in improving both your sperm health and your overall health. All of my patients who followed the recommendations contained in this chapter, experienced improved sperm health within three months.

Nutrients and Supplements

Many of the same nutrients and supplements that are beneficial for egg health, as described in the previous chapter, are also helpful for sperm health. In addition, just as in females and egg health, mitochondria, free radicals, and immune function play major roles in males and sperm health. Free radicals are among the by-products of mitochondrial energy production. If you don't have enough antioxidants to deal with the free radicals, this can result in damage to the sperm or eggs.

The following summarizes some of the studies that have reported benefits for sperm parameters. These summaries are simplified. As with the studies described in the previous chapter, if you are interested in reading more details about this research, please refer to the cited references.

CoQ10

CoQ10 (coenzyme Q10) is found in measurable levels in male seminal fluid (the fluid surrounding the sperm), and it likely has both antioxidant and metabolic functions. The concentration of CoQ10 has been shown to be directly correlated with both sperm count and sperm motility. In a study of men with low motility and low CoQ10 level, researchers found that if the men improved their CoQ10 levels, their sperm motility also improved[25].

In a study of men with oligoasthenoteratozoospermia (OAT), the tongue-twisting name for low sperm count and poor motility, researchers monitored sperm parameters as well as an enzyme called superoxide dismutase (SOD), which can degrade free radicals. The men received either CoQ10 (200 mg daily) or placebo for three months. Results showed that the men receiving the CoQ10 had improved sperm parameters and antioxidant status, compared with the placebo group[26].

Because CoQ10 can help with both mitochondrial function and free-radical neutralization, it can be a great supplement to support sperm count, motility, and morphology.

L-carnitine

As previously noted, L-carnitine is an amino acid that helps fatty-acid fuel enter mitochondria, allowing these organelles to produce energy. L-carnitine can play a significant role in supporting sperm motility. In a study evaluating seven randomized, controlled trials using L-carnitine in men with OAT, the researchers found significantly increased rates of spontaneous pregnancy and improved sperm motility in the L-carnitine groups compared to the control group. These positive results were noted with supplementation lasting between 12 and 26 weeks, but no significant changes in sperm counts or semen volume were noted[27].

Another study looked at using L-carnitine in men for only two weeks, leading up to an ICSI procedure. There were documented improvements in sperm motility and count, and more embryos developed in ICSI, for the L-carnitine group compared to the control group. The researchers concluded that short-term use of L-carnitine can improve sperm quality and increase the success rate of ICSI[28]. L-carnitine is generally dosed at 1 to 3 g/day to help with sperm quality.

NAC

N-acetylcysteine (NAC), as a reminder, is a building block for an antioxidant made by the liver called glutathione. There are studies showing that NAC can improve sperm parameters by enhancing antioxidant status in men with idiopathic (of unknown cause) infertility. In a study of 120 men with idiopathic infertility, half of the men received NAC (600 mg/day) and half received a placebo. The NAC group showed significant improvements in sperm motility and semen volume and viscosity, compared with the placebo group. However, there were no significant differences in sperm count or morphology between the two groups[29].

Zinc

Zinc is a mineral that plays an important role in immune function and as an antioxidant. Your body needs to maintain a balance between zinc and another mineral called copper. When this balance is upset, there can be major health consequences.

In a study of fertile males, the men were divided into four groups—those with low and high environmental exposure to copper and those with low and high environmental exposure to zinc. Semen/sperm volume, pH, count, motility, and morphology were monitored in all groups. The group with higher zinc exposure had significantly better results for progressively motile sperm (sperm that swim forward), as well as lower levels of an immune marker. The researchers concluded that zinc enhances sperm motility in fertile men, and that this improvement may be due to zinc reducing free radicals and modulating the immune system. Zinc is usually dosed at 30 to 50 mg/day, in a citrate or picolinate form[30].

Vitamin B12 and Folate

Vitamin B12 is important in cellular replication and the synthesis of DNA and RNA (ribonucleic acid). A lower B12 status has been associated with decreased sperm count and motility[31]. In one study, supplementation with a form of B12 called methylcobalamin (1,500 μg/day) in infertile men for 8 to 60 weeks resulted in significant improvements in sperm parameters[32]. In another study, vitamin B12 administration (1,000 μg/day) in men with lower sperm counts profoundly improved their counts at the end of 6 months of therapy[33].

Abnormal folate metabolism is an important factor contributing to male infertility[34]. Folic acid supplemented at 5 mg/day for 26 weeks improved sperm concentration, but not sperm motility or morphology, in one study[35]. Folic acid supplementation also has been shown to substantially improve pregnancy rates after assisted conception treatment[36].

Based on a wealth of research, diet and lifestyle factors play major roles in the health of sperm. The big take-home that I want to emphasize is that the healthier your sperm are at the time of conception, the healthier your baby will be.

Assignments

- Start implementing the changes described in the lifestyle section to improve your sperm health.

- If you have had a semen analysis and any of the parameters were not optimal, consider adding some of the supplements that we have discussed, depending on the particular issues raised by your analysis results.

- You can visit https://enhancefertility.ca/ for more info on sperm quality

CHAPTER 14
THE POWER OF POSITIVE THOUGHT AND VISUALIZATION

THE PROCESS OF getting pregnant comes easily to some, without requiring much thought. But for a considerable number of couples, pregnancy can become an extremely stressful issue. For these couples, it is important to understand the power of the mind and how having a positive mindset, with a focus on optimistic thoughts, can aid in your journey.

The monthly ups and downs that come with fertility struggles can take a huge toll on the psyche. I don't in any way want to minimize the pain and heartache that result from a failed cycle or miscarriage. These are events that can be traumatic, and losses need to be mourned and not brushed off. There are many fertility-focused mental-health therapists who can help couples develop coping strategies.

To assist couples in working through the setbacks and continuing on their fertility journey, incorporating certain techniques to help focus on the end goal and the positive wins along the way can be very helpful. In this chapter, you will learn to encourage your body to achieve your desired outcomes by following these strategies:

- Overcoming negative thoughts
- Promoting positive thoughts
- Incorporating visualization

"The power of positive thought" may sound like unimportant fluff, but there is actually a substantial amount of research showing that your thoughts directly impact both your physical and mental health. Your thoughts and attitudes also play significant roles in the health of your relationship.

Negative Thoughts

Let's begin by discussing the impact that negative thoughts can have on your body and on your mindset. Imagine that you are walking through the forest and you come across a bear in the middle of your path. The first thought that would likely come to mind is fear, and your body's response would be to run. Our brains are wired for immediate survival. When you have a negative thought like this, your mind will automatically shut out other thoughts or options to focus on survival. In this example, perhaps you could have climbed a tree or attempted to scare the bear as alternative actions, but your brain is hardwired for an automatic immediate response.

This is the case with all our negative emotions. Once a negative thought enters your mind, it can trigger strong emotions, like stress, anger, or fear. This emotion will then cause your mind to limit your ability to respond thoughtfully—your options become narrowed and you cannot think outside this hardwired pathway.

In our modern world, this phenomenon often occurs when you get into an argument and become so angry that you can't think rationally. Another example is when you feel so stressed or overwhelmed that you can't get anything done. In such cases, we often end up saying or doing something that we don't really intend. When the negative thoughts take hold, we usually lose our ability for rational thought and rely purely on instinct.

Positive Thoughts

When we have positive thoughts, by contrast, our mind is allowed to be open to multiple experiences and outcomes. Positive emotions - which can include joy, contentment, and love - allow your body to learn new skills that will persist long into the future. When you experience these emotions, it is easier for you to see different possibilities and options.

Countless studies have been conducted on optimism and positive thoughts. Almost all of them have come to the same conclusion. Optimistic people are healthier people. This has been shown to be true for physical health, with studies showing reductions in heart disease and improved immune function[37]. It has also been shown to be true for mental health, with less perceived stress, anxiety, and depression. Some studies have even suggested that women who are more optimistic have healthier babies and children[38].

For those of you who are used to thinking negative or pessimistic thoughts, don't worry. You can change. Optimism and positive thinking can be a learned skill. Following, are several guidelines to start changing your approach to situations:

1. Talk or think to yourself in a positive and kind way.

- Give yourself permission and encouragement to find something positive in any situation you find yourself in. For example, you wake up one morning to find it is -25°C (13°F) and sunny outside. Instead of focusing on the fact it is freezing cold, enjoy the fact that you have beautiful sunlight streaming through your windows.

- For some people, speaking to themselves out loud is extremely helpful for re-enforcing positive thoughts.

- Positive affirmations that are repeated daily will eventually become hardwired into your thought processes. They allow you to erase previously negative thoughts. Try adding a positive affirmation to anything you may be having doubts about. Examples of positive affirmations include:

    o I trust my body.
    o My hormones are in perfect balance.
    o A healthy egg is being developed.
    o My body is ready and knows how to conceive a healthy baby.

2. Avoid negative thought and self-talk.

    - Many people convince themselves that outcomes will be negative before they even attempt to start an endeavor. For example, if you wake up and tell yourself this is going to be a horrible day, it likely will be, because your mind will seek out the negative elements in all your experiences that day.

- For some people, stopping negative thoughts can be very challenging. There are several books and websites that can help you shift your outlook.
- The website "The Pursuit of Happiness" (http://www.pursuit-of-happiness.org/) is a non-profit science-based resource and online course that can help you learn to be more optimistic.

3. Think your way to success.

   - Research shows that, in general, successful people have more optimistic thoughts related to both health and wealth. You can choose how to react to situations that you are presented with in your life. You can choose to find the good in a situation or take on the role of victim. When you are a victim, you lose the ability to learn and find alternative outcomes, because you stay stuck within the negative single-track survival mode.

4. Take action every day.

   - If you can make small changes every day that keep you on track to achieve your goal, you will eventually get there. It will take a different amount of time for each person. Starting with simple behaviours that you repeat daily will allow those behaviours to develop into habits. Habits are a regular part of daily life, like brushing your teeth, exercising and choosing healthy foods. The accumulation of small changes over time will allow you to achieve your goals. Starting with a daily gratitude practice is a great way to start this. This could involve writing in a gratitude journal or expressing gratitude to loved ones or co-workers.

5. Set your expectations high.
   - If you never expect good things to happen to you, you will likely miss them when they do happen. It is helpful to adhere to the belief that your best days are ahead of you, rather than behind you. If you can't adopt this belief, it will be difficult to live your life to your maximum potential.

Visualization

Visualization can be a powerful tool to help calm your mind and body and to help you achieve your goals. Visualization basically involves closing your eyes and picturing exactly what you want, as clearly as possible, with details being as specific as you can make them. This process combines nicely with positive thoughts. Key aspects of the visualization process are summarized in the following points:

- Visualization works because when you imagine yourself doing exactly what you want, you physiologically create neural patterns in your brain, just as if you had physically performed the action. In other words, the thought can stimulate the nervous system in the same way as the actual event.

- The process of visualizing something positive will reduce stress and anxiety, relax the mind, and improve your overall mood. These changes, in turn, lower your blood pressure and allow your body to function at full capacity.

- Visualization is about going to your happy place and truly feeling present there and experiencing it fully. This can be possible even for something that hasn't happened yet. For example, if your happy place includes holding

THE POWER OF POSITIVE THOUGHT AND VISUALIZATION

your hoped-for baby, then see, hear, smell, touch, and feel the baby and everything else associated with you holding the baby, as if it all is actually happening at that moment.

- The key is to firmly believe that what you are visualizing is truly happening, and you need to really feel the experience.

- After a while, it will become increasingly easy to go to that happy place. When you do, you will find that worries diminish quickly.

- Visualization can be especially useful after hearing disappointing news, such as negative results from a pregnancy test.

- Performing or rehearsing an event in the mind trains the mind and body, creating the neural patterns that teach our bodies to do exactly what we want them to do.

- If your ultimate goal is for your body to conceive, then rehearse the conception process in your mind. After you and your partner have made love, or during an IUI or IVF procedure, visualize every step of the process, from the time the sperm enters the body and penetrates the egg, to the time the embryo implants itself into the uterus.

Some people prefer to make a physical vision board to help with the visualization process. Characteristics of vision boards include the following:

- A vision board is a collection of images and notes attached to a board and placed in a location where you can see it every day.

- The board should include a collage of images, phrases, poems, and quotes representing things that you would like to experience more in your life.
- The board serves as a visual representation of all the things that you want to do, be, and have in your life.
- The board is powerful because your attention is powerful. Where your attention goes, your energy flows. So, your attention should be focused on the things that you want to attract in your life.
- You can use vision boards for any aspect of your life.

In summary, practicing a combination of optimism, positive thinking, and visualization/vision boards will go a long way toward helping to improve both your physical health and mental health. Moreover, this will help to optimize your fertility.

Assignments

- Choose a few short positive phrases that you can repeat to yourself during the day to help develop your hard-wired neural pathways.
- Begin the visualization process by practicing with one or two scenarios that you want to see happen in your life. Try to engage all of your senses in your visualizations to make them feel as realistic as possible.
- Try creating a vision board to see if this approach is beneficial for you.

CHAPTER 15
STAYING CONNECTED AND OVERCOMING STRAIN ON RELATIONSHIPS

WORRIES, CONCERNS, AND problems that arise during the process of fertility treatment can put a great deal of strain on relationships. This applies to the relationship between partners, as well as relationships with friends, family members, and co-workers. This chapter focuses on:

- The importance of staying connected in your relationships throughout the fertility process
- Ways to reconnect with your partner if concerns develop

The Importance of Staying Connected or Reconnecting

When fertility problems arise in a relationship, it can be easy to retreat and close yourself off from your partner. This is more likely to happen if one partner feels that he or she is to blame. Fertility concerns can cause stress, not only to individuals, but to a marriage as well. When you are busy with tests, fertility charting, timed intercourse, and various medical procedures, a couple can stop connecting deeply like they once did.

It takes a lot of effort to stay open with each other emotionally and sexually. Nevertheless, making the effort will help keep your relationship intact through the challenging time you're both experiencing. Keeping in touch with your partner on an emotional level, through both nonsexual and sexual communication, becomes extremely important when you are trying to conceive. Feeling more connected to your partner will increase your feeling of comfort and reduce your stress levels and feeling of loneliness

Nonverbal connection through the eyes is especially valuable in creating a deep and lasting connection, not just with your partner, but with other loved ones and friends as well.

Connecting Through the Eyes

One of the best techniques for connecting is eye-gazing. The experience of looking your partner in the eyes can change the tone of your interactions. Looking away from your partner does a great disservice to both of you.

Eye-gazing originated in our prehistoric primate days, so this is nothing new. It has always been a way that men and women flirt, connect, and get each other's attention.

When you and your partner first fell in love, there was most likely an exciting, passionate attraction between the two of you. You probably wanted to touch and look at each other all the time. As your relationship developed, especially through the stresses of trying to conceive, those intense feelings probably tended to fade. But they are not gone. You just need to put in a little more effort to bring them back to the surface.

Eye-gazing provides a way to connect and communicate with your partner that is completely nonverbal. It helps build a strong connection with powerful emotions that activate a hormonal response that prepares your bodies for conception. Regularly engaging in eye-gazing may be challenging at first, but the payoff can be profound for you and your partner.

Benefits of Eye-Gazing

There are many wonderful benefits of eye-gazing that go beyond connecting with your partner. Looking people in the eye allows you to connect with anyone you meet, making them feel like you care. But can you remember the last time someone truly looked you in the eye when he or she spoke to you? It has become a lost art. With the advent of modern technology, we now often communicate electronically instead of face-to-face. Today, it is common to see two people out together and both are busy with their cell phones—not present with each other at all.

Those people are missing the benefits of eye-gazing. These benefits include the following:

- Connecting through the eyes can increase your self-esteem and make you feel more confident.

- Eye-gazing will keep you focused on the present moment, rather than worrying about all the other things going on in your life.

- It helps build trust. Having greater trust leads to better, more exhilarating sex.

- It deepens your emotional connection. A number of scientific studies have shown that consistent eye contact is one of the best ways to bond with your partner.
- Eye-gazing during sex can be extremely arousing. It's an amazing experience to watch your partner experience pleasure, and to watch him or her be a witness to your own pleasure.
- By allowing yourself to gaze into the eyes of another person and simply breathe—relaxing all thought and being fully present—you will experience a deep sense of connection and love.
- This practice alone can help you feel more supported throughout your fertility journey.

Although it seems like a basic behavior, eye-gazing may require practice to perform effectively. The following guidelines will help you develop your eye-gazing skills:

- Practice gazing into your partner's eyes for two or three minutes. In this exercise, you may feel uncomfortable, exposed, and even afraid. Resist the urge to look away when confronted with these thoughts and emotions. Allow your thoughts and emotions to pass, as they certainly will, until they give way to an inner peacefulness and calm.
- Start eye-gazing with your partner in lower-intensity situations, such as when you're talking about your day. Work your way up to making contact during more vulnerable moments, such as when you're sharing your feelings.
- During eye-gazing, you should relax your eyes. You need not stare, and you shouldn't worry about blinking.

- (This isn't a contest!) Blinking is good, and having a soft gaze is more effective.
- As you make eye contact, sit or lay across from each other and begin to breathe comfortably. With each breath, allow yourself to become more and more open and comfortable connecting with each other.
- Allow the process to unfold slowly. You may notice that you begin to feel much more unified with your partner.
- After your initial eye-gazing exercises, you can allow the process to go wherever you choose to take it. When you both feel ready, try making eye contact when you or your partner are initiating sex, or during sex. Notice how this practice changes the energy between the two of you.

Assignments

- This week spend time each day connecting with your partner. Practice gazing into your partner's eyes for a couple minutes while you are talking with each other. This can happen at any time during the day—in the morning over breakfast, when you get home from work, or before bed. Also try, at least once, to spend a couple minutes gazing into each other's eyes without speaking.
- Practice making eye contact with other people with whom you speak, besides your partner. This could be people at work, at family gatherings, at the grocery store, or anywhere else.
- Make note of the differences that eye-contact makes in your relationships, as well as in the way you feel about yourself and other people.

CHAPTER 16
THE ROLE OF HORMONE-DISRUPTING TOXINS IN FERTILITY

THERE ARE THOUSANDS of different kinds of toxins in our environment. Each day, we are exposed to hundreds of toxins, several of which can have a negative impact on our health. One class of toxins called hormone disruptors, or endocrine disruptors, can play a large role in causing problems with fertility and reproductive health. In this chapter, we will discuss the following issues regarding hormone disruptors:

- Where these types of toxins occur
- Ways to reduce your exposure to these toxins
- How to improve your body's ability to eliminate these toxins

THE ROLE OF HORMONE-DISRUPTING TOXINS IN FERTILITY

Overview of Hormone Disruptors

The Environmental Working Group (EWG), the non-profit environmental protection group that we mentioned in a previous chapter, published the following list of the 12 most common hormone-disrupting chemicals[39]:

- Bisphenol A (BPA)
- Dioxin
- Atrazine
- Phthalates
- Perchlorate
- Fire retardants
- Lead
- Mercury
- Arsenic
- Perfluorinated chemicals (PFCs)
- Organophosphate pesticides
- Glycol ethers

We are exposed to the majority of these chemicals daily. Some are easier to avoid than others. Common places where these toxins can be found include lotions, makeup, soaps and detergents, household cleaning products, yard-care products, food-storage containers, and the water supply. This list is not meant to make you panic, but to increase your awareness of the chemical exposures that you can minimize.

How do these toxins cause hormonal problems? Some of these chemicals bind to the same cellular receptors that your hormones bind to. This "tricks" your body into "thinking" that you have either more or fewer circulating hormones than you actually have, disrupting metabolic processes that depend on hormonal balance. Other hormone-disrupting chemicals increase or decrease the amounts of certain hormones that your body secretes. Still others mimic the function of the hormones. The main concern with all these compounds is that the levels of certain hormones will change in your body, and this can lead to changes in menstrual cycle, impair the ability of the thyroid to function properly, and impact how the body responds to stress. Some of these compounds are linked to specific conditions that reduce reproductive ability. For example, phthalates are associated with endometriosis, which adversely impacts a woman's ability to conceive. Hormone disruptors have also been linked to breast and reproductive cancers, early puberty, heart disease, obesity, and other conditions.

Laboratory tests are available to determine the levels of various hormone-disrupting chemicals in your body. For example, to test for such toxic metals as lead and mercury, the best assessment is a pre- and post-provocation urinalysis. This test involves collecting a sample of urine first thing in the morning, then taking a so-called provoking agent (such as dimercaptosuccinic acid-DMSA), and six hours later collecting a second urine sample. Analysis of the first urine sample reveals if you have current ongoing exposures to toxic metals. Analysis of the second urine sample indicates how much toxic metal is stored in your tissues. If high concentrations are detected, you should get detoxification treatment before trying to conceive. This is especially important with lead, which is mainly stored in bone. During pregnancy, due to your body's heavy use of calcium, you experience rapid turnover of bone tissue. If there are high levels of lead in your bones, this toxin can pass directly through the placenta to your growing baby.

There are also tests available for other toxic chemicals, including pesticides, insecticides, and plastic compounds.

To learn more about this testing, you should consult your health provider.

Minimizing Exposure

Toxins are so ubiquitous in the environment that you can never completely eliminate your exposure to them. You can, however, take actions to minimize your exposure and encourage your body to eliminate and excrete the toxins instead of storing them. The following focuses on three toxic compounds from the EWG list that are relatively easy to avoid yet can have significant impact on fertility. These compounds are BPA, phthalates, and mercury.

1. BPA is a chemical compound that is used to make epoxy resins, which are found in some food-storage containers, and polycarbonates, which are found in many items made of hard plastic. Inside the body, BPA imitates estrogen. One study detected BPA in 9 out of 10 samples of umbilical cord blood, so we know it passes through the placenta to the baby. Ways to minimize exposure to BPA include:

    - Use fewer canned foods and use more fresh foods, because most metal-lined food containers contain BPA. Note, however, those food products that are labeled "BPA-free."

    - Avoid hard-plastic food containers, especially those with labels indicating polycarbonate (PC) or recycling symbol 7. These items often contain BPA.

    - Never microwave food in plastic containers. The heating of plastic can cause BPA to leach into the food.

- If you don't need receipts with your purchases, avoid taking them. The thermal paper used in register machines is often coated with BPA. BPA has been widely recognized as a hormone disruptor, and policies have been enacted in Canada and the United States to remove this substance from a variety of products, including baby bottles. Some manufacturers have taken it upon themselves to remove BPA from their plastic products, and such products are usually labeled "BPA-free".

2. Phthalates are one of the most serious concerns when it comes to reproductive health. These chemicals have been linked to thyroid irregularities, diabetes, lower sperm counts and less mobile sperm.

    To reduce your exposure to phthalates, look at the ingredients in your personal care products. Phthalates are usually listed in the ingredients as "fragrance." You will also find these chemicals in most plastic food containers, some children's toys, and plastic wrap made from polyvinyl chloride (PVC) or labeled with recycling symbol 3. Phthalates have been banned from some children's products.

    A great resource for checking the toxicity of your personal care products is the EWG page titled "EWG's Skin Deep Cosmetics Database," which can be found at www.ewg.org/skindeep.

3. Mercury is a naturally occurring metal that is toxic to human health. Mercury exposure can have a major impact on reproduction, because it binds directly to hormones regulating the menstrual cycle and ovulation. This interferes with proper hormonal signaling. Mercury gets into the air and water from many different

activities, including emissions from coal-fired power plants. Our most common exposure to mercury is through the consumption of larger fish. Tuna and swordfish have some of the highest levels of mercury. Therefore, you should avoid eating these fish when pregnant or trying to conceive.

The Body's Elimination of Toxins

Although we cannot completely avoid exposure to all toxins, our bodies have natural ways of eliminating at least some of the toxins to which we are exposed. One of the most effective ways is sweating. Sweating can best be promoted through exercise or through use of a sauna. Ideally, if you are going to use a sauna, do so after exercise. During exercise, your body will use its stored glycogen, or sugar, reserves. Once you have used up these sugars, your body will start burning fat as a fuel source. Many of the hormone-disrupting chemicals get stored in your fat cells. So, when you start using fat as a fuel source, some of those toxins will start circulating. The more you are sweating, the more these toxins will get eliminated through your sweat.

Keep in mind that with prolonged sweating, you need to ensure that you rehydrate properly to keep your electrolytes balanced. Make sure that you drink enough water to keep your urine pale yellow to clear. Furthermore, ensuring proper hydration is crucial for your body's ability to continually deal with the toxin exposures you are bombarded with daily.

The body's other routes of detoxification include the digestive system, liver and kidney functions, and lymphatic activity. These routes can be optimized by certain behaviors. In terms of digestive health, it is important to have at least two bowel movements daily. Movements should be easy to pass, in a log shape, and not contain blood or mucous. If this is not the way your digestive system is currently working, you might have foods in your diet that are creating inflammation in your digestive system and, potentially, in the rest of your body. Certain foods promote digestive detoxification. For example, root vegetables—including beets, sweet potatoes, yams, and parsnips—will assist the liver in functioning more efficiently. Including these vegetables in your diet will be helpful in boosting your body's ability to move toxins out.

Assignments

- Start reducing your exposure to hormone-disrupting chemicals. Check the ingredients in your personal care products as the first step. Toxic products are easy to replace with non-toxic alternatives.

- Work on optimizing your routes of elimination. Perform an activity at least four days per week that makes you sweat substantially. If you have access to a sauna, try to use it on a regular basis.

- Remember that reducing the level of toxicity in your body will help to rebalance your hormonal system and improve your chances of getting pregnant.

- Looking for support and suggestions on reducing toxin exposures you can join the Facebook group Enhance Fertility

CHAPTER 17
GENES AND FERTILITY

EVERY PERSON HAS a unique set of genes—or genome—that contains instructions for the way his or her body looks and the way it functions. Some genes influence your fertility and other reproductive processes. Some genes increase your risk of getting certain diseases. However, not all of these genetic instructions are "set in stone." Environmental factors—such as the foods you eat, the chemicals you are exposed to, and the medications you take—can influence the activity and expression of genes. These factors may be able to essentially turn certain genes "on" or "off." Thus, there are ways to optimizing your genetic potential to improve your chances of becoming a parent.

This chapter will shed light on the following points:

- How your genes impact your fertility and pregnancy
- How your genes affect the health of your baby
- What you can do to influence the activity of your genes

Genetic Basics

The genes you inherited from your mother and father allow you to share certain traits with them and other family members. But, on a basic level, how does this genetic process work?

During conception, you inherit two copies of each of your genes, one from each parent. Your particular collection of genes makes up your individual genome (or genotype). There are approximately 20,000 genes in the human genome. Each gene is made of a unique sequence of four nucleotide building blocks, known as adenine (A), cytosine (C), guanine (G), and thymine (T). These building blocks form so-called bases, which pair with one another (A with T, C with G) along the double-stranded DNA molecules. Genes range in size from hundreds of base pairs to more than 2 million base pairs. Human genes are further arranged into 23 pairs of chromosomes. Each cell of your body contains these chromosomes.

During the process of cellular reproduction, changes can sometimes occur at certain points in the sequence of nucleotides (A, C, G, T) in the genes. When there is a single letter that changes, this is known as a single nucleotide polymorphism (SNP). SNPs are the most common type of genetic change, or mutation, that happens in humans. They are passed from parent to offspring. Different SNPs will have different impacts on the ways that genes behave—the genes' instructions for the body. There are some SNPs that affect your body's ability to prevent free radicals from damaging your eggs or sperm. Other SNPs influence how your body processes hormones and toxins. Still others influence how your body responds to medications.

Knowing your genotype, including the types of SNPs in your cells, can help you determine if you will respond well to a particular medication, and it could indicate why you respond differently than some other people to certain substances, such as alcohol or caffeine. Knowing if you have a particular

SNP will help you understand how the gene may work for you, allowing you to personalize your treatments and lifestyle choices based on your individual genetic legacy.

There are several companies that offer genome testing that could reveal many types of SNPs, including those that affect fertility. If you use such testing services, you should get the results interpreted by a trained healthcare professional who understands the implications of genes in fertility.

The remarkable thing about SNPs is their ability to essentially be turned on, turned off, or dimmed. Expression of an SNP can change based on diet, supplement use, and lifestyle changes. Once you have been able to optimize your choices based on your genetic individuality, you may notice that some health problems will start to lessen or even disappear. In my clinical practice, I have often found that patients who have unexplained infertility, PCOS, or endometriosis see considerable improvements after making lifestyle adjustments based on their SNP profiles.

Three Important SNPs

In the following, I focus on three SNPs that play major roles in fertility.

1. **MTHFR (Methylenetetrahydrofolate Reductase)**

    MTHFR is a gene involved in the detoxification pathway called methylation. This gene allows your body to make an enzyme that converts folate into its active form, 5-MTHFR, which is used in multiple metabolic processes. If you don't have a favorable SNP version for this gene, your body has reduced ability to convert folate into a useable form and to detoxify itself. These processes are important for the repair and synthesis of DNA and for metabolism involving hormones and neurotransmitters. Metabolic problems can lead to mood concerns, hormonal imbalance, and poor development of both eggs and sperm. If folate is not properly converted to its active form, high levels of an amino acid called homocysteine can contribute to cardiovascular disease, including high blood pressure and stroke. Proper folate conversion is also essential for the early stages of fetal development and for the prevention of birth defects.

The MTHFR gene can have two Ts, two Cs, or one of each. If you have two Cs, the gene is able to work with optimal function, and consumption of a healthy diet would be expected to allow normal function of the MTHFR enzyme. If you have one C and one T, your MTHFR enzyme will work at about 65 percent the efficiency (or rate) of someone with two Cs. This means that with good lifestyle habits, you would likely not notice the diminished enzyme capacity. However, if you are experiencing mood, hormonal, or cardiovascular problems, you may need a folate supplement. During preconception and early pregnancy, supplementing with an active folate called L-5-MTHFR would help ensure that your body is getting enough active folate.

If you have two Ts in the MTHFR gene, your MTHFR enzyme will work at only about 20 percent to 30 percent the efficiency of someone with two Cs[40]. I have found that many patients with depression, anxiety, ADHD, or a history of recurrent miscarriage have two Ts. For these patients, I generally recommend avoiding fortified grains for at least three months and supplementing with active L-5-MTHFR folate before trying to conceive. Fortified grains contain synthetic folic acid. If patients with two Ts consume synthetic folic acid, it increases the potential for early miscarriage in females and poor sperm quality in males or birth defects[41].

2. **CYP 1A2 (Cytochrome P450 1A2)**

   The detoxification pathway through the liver is separated into two phases. In the first phase (phase 1), the liver takes substances such as estrogens, certain medications, caffeine, alcohol or other toxins, and changes the makeup of the substances to isolate the most toxic parts. In the second phase (phase 2), the liver identifies the toxins formed in phase 1 and works to clear them from the body. The eliminated substances are carcinogenic or pro-inflammatory in nature. If both phases of this process are working well, you are likely eliminating these toxins effectively. If the phases are not working well, you will see the development of symptoms associated with poor detoxification and poor elimination. In terms of hormone-related problems, these symptoms may include flare-ups of endometriosis, acne or other skin changes, fatigue, and mental fog.

   The CYP 1A2 gene is responsible for the metabolic speed of phase 1. This gene can have two As, two Gs, or one of each. If you have two As, you are a fast metabolizer. This is not good, because phase 1 will proceed too quickly. If phase 2 cannot keep up with the fast metabolism of phase 1, you may accumulate toxins that cause inflammation or DNA damage (and possibly cancer) before they are eliminated from the body. Fast metabolizers are at higher risk of miscarriage with caffeine intake[42]. You can slow down phase 1 by using certain herbs, such as curcumin. This will help to counteract the inflammatory and carcinogenic effects of fast metabolism.

If you have one G or two Gs in the CYP 1A2 gene, you are a slow metabolizer, which is ideal for phase 1. In these cases, no lifestyle modification is needed.

3. **SOD2 (Superoxide Dismutase 2)**

    SOD2 is a gene that codes for an enzyme that promotes oxidative phosphorylation inside your mitochondria. These organelles, as a reminder, are responsible for producing energy in the cells of your body. Oxidative phosphorylation helps to prevent free radicals from damaging mitochondria. This is particularly relevant to fertility, because mitochondria play a crucial role in the healthy development of your eggs and sperm, as well as in the development of the blastocyst once conception has taken place. Mitochondria provide the energy necessary for all of these processes. If mitochondria can't produce adequate amounts of energy, conception is unlikely.

    The SOD2 gene can have two Ts, two Cs, or one of each. The two-C genotype is associated with optimal function of the SOD2 enzyme. The two-T genotype is associated with a 10-fold higher risk of heart disease, as well as with other inflammatory processes. Furthermore, this genotype can be a major contributor to poor egg and sperm quality. If you have two Ts and are struggling with fertility, it is imperative that you minimize your exposure to free radicals and increase your consumption of antioxidants, either through foods or supplements[43].

Summary

Many of our genes work in conjunction with one another, so they cannot be interpreted on their own, but rather in groupings. This chapter serves as a simple introduction to genomics and speaks to a few SNPs that play roles in fertility. There are several additional SNPs that come into play in fertility issues. However, you should now be aware that you can modulate the effects of your genes through diet, supplementation, medications, or other lifestyle changes.

Understanding your genetic legacy will go a long way toward helping you choose the most effective lifestyle changes for yourself. Your genes hold the key to your future, for both disease prevention and individualized medicine to optimize your health and fertility.

Assignments

- Have you ever had a personal genome analysis? If so, did you learn anything about your health- or fertility-related genes? Were you able to apply this information to benefit your health?

- If you have never had a personal genome analysis, conduct some online research into these services. Focus on those that are health-related. Also ask your healthcare provider about these services. After you collect sufficient information, consider using one of the services. What type of information would you hope to learn about your genes? How would you apply this information to your health?

FINAL THOUGHTS

I realize that there is a large amount of information throughout this book and that it may be a lot to take in. If you are feeling overwhelmed, try reading and implementing the suggestions one chapter a week until they become routine. This approach will help the changes feel comfortable and provide you with a great sense of accomplishment. Make sure to celebrate the small victories along the way.

I know that it can sometimes feel as though everyone around you is pregnant, and there are times when you will struggle with why it isn't happening for you as well. Keep in mind that about one in six couples have difficulty conceiving, so please know that you are never alone and you are not the only one going through this.

If you feel that you would benefit from individualized support please reach out. We can offer one or one consultations email info@enhancefertility.ca. You can visit the website at: https://enhancefertility.ca/ to sign up for our newsletter with the latest updates in fertility research. You can follow us on social media at @enhancefertility on either Facebook or Instagram.

ENDNOTES

1. Van Die MD, et al. Vitex agnus-castus extracts for female reproductive disorders: a systematic review of clinical trials. *Planta Med.* 2013 May;79(7):562-75

2. Liang Y, et al. Villainous role of estrogen in macrophage-nerve interaction in endometriosis. *Reprod Biol Endocrinol.* 2018 Dec 5;16(1):122.

3. Zhu Y, et al. Prevalent genotypes of methylenetetrahydrofolate reductase (MTHFR) in recurrent miscarriage and recurrent implantation failure. *J Assist Reprod Genet.* 2018 Aug;35(8):1437-1442.

4. Bharwani A, et al. Oral treatment with Lactobacillus rhamnosus attenuates behavioural deficits and immune changes in chronic social stress. *BMC Med.* 2017 Jan 11;15(1):7.

5   Baker EJ, et al. Metabolism and functional effects of plant-derived omega-3 fatty acids in humans. *Prog Lipid Res.* 2016 Oct;64:30-56

6   Franasiak JM, et al. Vitamin D in human reproduction. *Curr Opin Obstet Gynecol.* 2017 Aug;29(4):189-194

7   Pal L, et al. Vitamin D status relates to reproductive outcome in women with polycystic ovary syndrome: secondary analysis of a multicentre randomized controlled trial. *J. clin. Endocrinol metab.* 2016;101:3027-3035

8   Ben-Meir A, et al. Coenzyme Q10 restores oocyte mitochondrial function and fertility during reproductive aging. *Aging Cell.* 2015 Oct;14(5):887-95.

9   Kitano Y, et al. Oral administration of l-carnitine improves the clinical outcome of fertility in patients with IVF treatment. *Gynecol Endocrinol.* 2018 Aug;34(8):684-688.

10 Bennett M. Vitamin B12 deficiency, infertility and recurrent fetal loss. *J Reprod Med.* 2001 Mar;46(3):209-12.

11 Vujkovic M, et al. Associations between dietary patterns and semen quality in men undergoing IVF/ICSI treatment. *Hum Reprod.* 2009 Jun;24(6):1304-12.

12 Paffoni A, et al. Homocysteine pathway and in vitro fertilization outcome. *Reprod Toxicol.* 2018 Mar;76:12-16.

13 Chavarro JE, et al. Iron intake and risk of ovulatory infertility. *Obstet Gynecol.* 2006 Nov;108(5):1145-52.

14 Dastorani M, et al. The effects of vitamin D supplementation on metabolic profiles and gene expression of

ENDNOTES

insulin and lipid metabolism in infertile polycystic ovary syndrome candidates for in vitro fertilization. *Reprod Biol Endocrinol.* 2018 Oct 4;16(1):94.

15   Kuroda M, et al. Levothyroxine supplementation improves serum anti-Müllerian hormone levels in infertile patients with Hashimoto's thyroiditis. *J Obstet Gynaecol Res.* 2018 Apr;44(4):739-746.

16   https://www.apa.org/news/press/releases/stress/2017/state-nation.pdf

17   Russell J, et al. Daily protein content correlates with increased fertility and pregnancy outcome. ACOG 2013, Abstract poster

18   Vartanyan EV, et al. Improvement in quality of oocytes in polycystic ovarian syndrome in programs of in vitro fertilization. *Gynecol Endocrinol.* 2017;33 (sup1):8-11.

19   Artini PG, et al. Endocrine and clinical effects of myo-inositol administration in polycystic ovary syndrome. *Gynecol Endocrinol.* 2013;29(4):375-9.

20   Pacchiarotti A, et al. Effect of myo-inositol and melatonin versus myo-inositol, in a randomized controlled trial, for improving in vitro fertilization of patients with polycystic ovarian syndrome. *Gynecol Endocrinol.* 2016;32(1):69-73.

21   Rago R, et al. Effect of myo-inositol and alpha-lipoic acid on oocyte quality in polycystic ovary syndrome non-obese women undergoing in vitro fertilization: a pilot study. *J Biol Regul Homeost Agents.* 2015;29(4): 913-23.

22 Refaeey A, et al. Combined coenzyme Q10 and clomiphene citrate for ovulation in clomiphene-citrate-resistant polycystic ovary syndrome. *Reprod Biomed Online.* 2014;29(1):119-24.

23 Cheraghi E, et al. N-Acetylcysteine improves oocyte and embryo quality in polycystic ovary syndrome patients undergoing intracytoplasmic sperm injection: an alternative to metformin. *Reprod Fertil Dev.* 2016 Apr;28(6):723-31.

24 Giorgi VS, et al. N-acetyl-cysteine and L-carnitine prevent meiotic oocyte damage induced by follicular fluid from infertile women with mild endometriosis. *Reprod Sci.* 2016 Mar;23(3):342-51.

25 Balercia G, et al. Coenzyme Q10 treatment in infertile men with idiopathic asthenozoospermia: A placebo-controlled, double-blind randomized trial. *Fertility and Sterility.* 2009;91(5):1785–92.

26 Safarinejad MR, et al. Effects of the reduced form of coenzyme Q10 (ubiquinol) on semen parameters in men with idiopathic infertility: A double-blind, placebo controlled, randomized study. *The Journal of Urology.* 2012;188(2):526–31.

27 Shang XJ, et al. Effect and safety of L-carnitine in the treatment of idiopathic oligoasthenozoospermia: a systemic review. *Zhonghua Na Ke Xue.* 2015 Jan;21(1):65-73.

28 Wu ZM, et al. Short-term medication of L-carnitine before intracytoplasmic sperm injection for infertile men with oligoasthenozoospermia. *Zhonguna Nan Ke Xue.* 2012 Mar;18(3):253-6.

ENDNOTES

29 Ciftci H, et al. Effects of N-acetylcysteine on semen parameters and oxidative/antioxidant status. *Urology.* 2009;74(1):73–6.

30 Ahmadi S, et al. Antioxidant supplements and semen parameters: An evidence based review. *International Journal of Reproductive Biomedicine.* 2016;14(12):729–36.

31 Sinclair S. Male infertility: Nutritional and environmental considerations. *Alternative Medicine Review.* 2000;5(1):28–38.

32 Ahmadi S, et al. Antioxidant supplements and semen parameters: An evidence based review. *International Journal of Reproductive Biomedicine.* 2016;14(12):729–36.

33 Sandler B and B Faragher. Treatment of oligospermia with vitamin B12. *Infertility.* 1984;7:133–8.

34 Murphy LE, et al. Folate and vitamin B12 in idiopathic male infertility. *Asian Journal of Andrology.* 2011;13(6):856–61.

35 Wong WY, et al. Effects of folic acid and zinc sulfate on male factor subfertility: A double-blind, randomized, placebo-controlled trial. *Fertility and Sterility.* 2002;77(3):491–98.

36 Ahmadi S, et al. Antioxidant supplements and semen parameters: An evidence based review. *International Journal of Reproductive Biomedicine.* 2016;14(12):729–36.

37 Kim MY, et al. Relationship Between Types of Social Support, Coping Strategies, and Psychological Distress in Individuals Living With Congenital Heart Disease. *J Cardiovasc Nurs.* 2019 Jan/Feb;34(1):76-84

38 Castro-Schilo L, et al. Parents' Optimism, Positive Parenting, and Child Peer Competence in Mexican-Origin Families. *Parent Sci Pract.* 2013 Apr 1; 13(2): 95–112.

39 https://www.ewg.org/ Viewed December 10, 2018.

40 Merviel P, et al. Comparison of two preventive treatments for patients with recurrent miscarriages carrying a C677T methylenetetrahydrofolate reductase mutation: 5-year experience. *J Int Med Res.* 2017 Dec; 45(6): 1720–1730.

41 Jedidi L, et al. Autosomal single-gene disorders involved in human infertility. *Saudi J Biol Sci.* 2018 Jul;25(5):881-887

42 Sata F, et al. Caffeine intake, CYP1A2 polymorphism and the risk of recurrent pregnancy loss. *Mol Hum Reprod.* 2005 May;11(5):357-60.

43 Agarwal A, et al. Role of oxidative stress in female reproduction. *Reprod Biol Endocrinol.* 2005 Jul 14;3:28.

ABOUT THE AUTHOR

Dr. Jodie Peacock ND has a special interest in women's health, with a focus on hormone balancing and fertility. Dr. Peacock graduated from the University of Guelph and went on to complete 4 years of study at the Canadian College of Naturopathic medicine. After being diagnosed with polycystic ovarian syndrome (PCOS) in her early twenties, she concentrated on learning how to naturally optimize hormonal health. As a naturopathic doctor, and mother of three, she can attest to the positive impact which simple changes to diet and lifestyle can have on conception and children's health. Dr. Peacock is passionate about educating couples on how to optimize their fertility and is the Chief medical officer for Enhance Fertility https://enhancefertility.ca/ and founder of the Canadian Fertility Show www.canadianfertilityshow.ca.

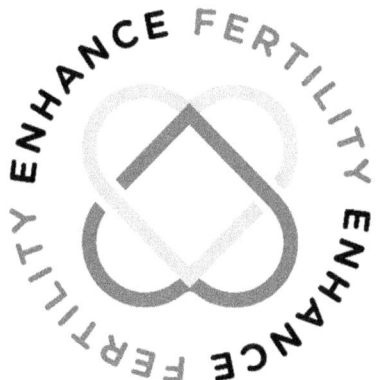

If you enjoyed reading Preconceived, I would highly encourage you to join the Enhance Fertility mailing list. Joining the mail list will give you a download of our fertility supportive recipe book.

As a thank you for reading Preconceived, we are offering readers a **15%** discount off the Enhance Fertility supplements. Please enter code Preconceived on the check out page to receive your discount.

https://enhancefertility.ca/

Any questions please email info@enhancefertility.ca

www.ingramcontent.com/pod-product-compliance
Lightning Source LLC
LaVergne TN
LVHW011838060526
838200LV00054B/4090